COOK. HEAL.

Go Vegan!

A Delicious Guide to
Plant-Based Cooking for Better Health
and a Better World

CHEF BAI

Bailey Ruskus

PAGE STREET
PUBLISHING CO.

PAGE STREET
PUBLISHING CO.

First published in 2021 by
Page Street Publishing Co.
27 Congress Street, Suite 105
Salem, MA 01970
www.pagestreetpublishing.com

Distributed by Macmillan, sales in Canada by The Canadian Manda Group.

25   24   23   22   21   1   2   3   4   5

ISBN-13: 978-1-64567-306-4
ISBN-10: 1-64567-306-5

Library of Congress Control Number: 2020948800

Cover and book design by Rosie Stewart for Page Street Publishing Co.
Photography by Bailey Ruskus

Printed and bound in China

For anyone who has ever been told they can't heal.

And for those who tried anyway.

And for my husband. This work wouldn't be here without your dedication to the mission and to us. I love you.

Contents

Introduction

We are living in a time in which we are redefining what it means to be vegan and in which realities about our world are changing so quickly, our actions must be louder than our words. Switching to a plant-based diet is one of the most powerful things you can do for your health and the world around you. It's a decision rooted in compassion for ourselves and the animals that walk this Earth alongside us. It's a way of life fueled by the desperate need for change in our world.

The reality is that we don't need a few people doing it perfectly, we need millions and millions of people trying their best and doing it imperfectly. Eating food that is grown, not raised. Cooking consciously and leaning into the incredible abundance that the plant world has to offer us. It's about embracing the self-healing powers of our bodies when they're given the right tools to heal.

I was trained at Le Cordon Bleu and spent the first six years of my professional cooking career in San Francisco. Even though I didn't learn much about veganism during my training and early culinary work, I learned a whole hell of a lot about cooking. I understood the importance of eating for joy and unapologetically seeking out pleasure for your meals: 3 meals a day, 365 days a year. I was also silently suffering with endometriosis and a debilitating daily dose of chronic pain to match. I ate food that would numb my pain, drank excessive amounts of alcohol and hopped on the hamster wheel like millions of other people—that is, the endless wheel of unhealthy food, prescriptions, pain, inflammation, alcohol and doctors' offices.

I felt that in order to experience pleasure in life, I also had to experience pain. A great example of that is the hangover you get after a fun night of drinking. Or was it actually the other way around? I was experiencing so much pain that the only way I could convince myself to get up and be a productive member of society was to fuel my easily accessible and quickly satisfied pleasure centers of cheese, pastries, meat and alcohol.

After years of living a life like this, I inevitably got tired. I started to do my own research, went back to school for nutrition and learned that there are millions of other people living and silently suffering like I was. Shortly after that, I discovered that my suffering was my biggest resource to create real change in my life and the world around me. I learned about the injustices of our food system, the health crisis Western society is in, the realities of animal agriculture and the negative effect all of this has on our environment. It seemed ridiculous to me that I had been asleep to all of it and had paid $100,000 for an education that had taught me so much but also allowed me to contribute so much more to all that suffering. The beauty of it all is that I learned how to do one thing really, really well. And that, my friend, is how to cook.

I discovered that my chef's knife was my best way to enact change in this world. To open the eyes of friends, family and strangers with incredible plant-based food. There's no need for the disclosure of, "It's vegan," because this food speaks for itself and can satisfy all humans. The disclosure is more of a, "Don't worry, I've got you." Plant-based food is rich in nutrients and not incredibly calorie-dense like its animal-based counterparts. This means that abundance is knocking on your door when you are on this plant-based journey. There's no need for obsessing about calories or feeling guilty for your meals. You can let go of the limiting bounds of a few main types of animal foods for your calories and gain the plant world, which has more than ten thousand edible varieties to choose from.

The most beautiful thing about this diet and lifestyle change is that I believe it has the power to save lives, and not just the lives of animals. With the help of the right team of doctors and healers who understand and listen to you, this lifestyle change has the potential to save you from endless prescriptions, depression, weight that doesn't belong to you and the all-too-common disconnect from our natural word. It can awaken something deep within you that helps food make sense in a way it never has before. And I'll tell you some encouraging news: You will actually start to heal.

In order to heal, we must first find our joy. A really easy way to find joy is to look to something that you do three times a day, every day. Cooking with vibrant, local and seasonal food can connect you back to the earth, back to yourself, and with the right tools, it can get you on a whole new vibe! Immersing yourself in farmers' markets and delicious recipes isn't just for chefs—it's something that appeals to your basic makeup as a human being and can reconnect you with yourself and, most importantly, your joy of cooking.

If you've been waiting for a sign, this is it. This book can help you take back your power. It can help you rediscover what it means to be human while bringing vibrancy back into your life. These recipes and concepts are fueled with purpose and intention so that you can heal, gain confidence in the kitchen and enjoy every single bite. There is no room for bland or boring "healthy food." There's no more time to wait for the next New Year's resolution to get started.

Your skin will start to glow, your body odor will change (in a good way!), you'll sleep deeper and your body will transform with less inflammation and less puffiness. The recipes in this book can help you achieve all of that while also avoiding food boredom. Hopefully, you can cook your way through this entire book. At the end of it, you will have a new and deeper connection to your kitchen and your relationship to food. I want you to create meals for your loved ones and to be proud of what you've created. You won't need to convince them to like it because it's good for them, as this delicious food speaks for itself.

Don't put a lot of pressure on yourself to be perfect. Just flow with it, find your joy and enjoy the process. These recipes are a guide to help you cook intuitively. Many of them are simple ideas with classic techniques that are supported by big purpose and even bigger flavors.

Remember, we are all in this together. Something inspired you to pick up this book, and I hope these words inspire you to flip the page, grab your chef's knife and continue this journey through the realm of your kitchen. If you're totally new to cooking or to plant-based eating, or if you're a twenty-year vegan or a professional chef looking for a new way, this book was written for you. The beginner's mindset can truly help us cook, heal and go vegan.

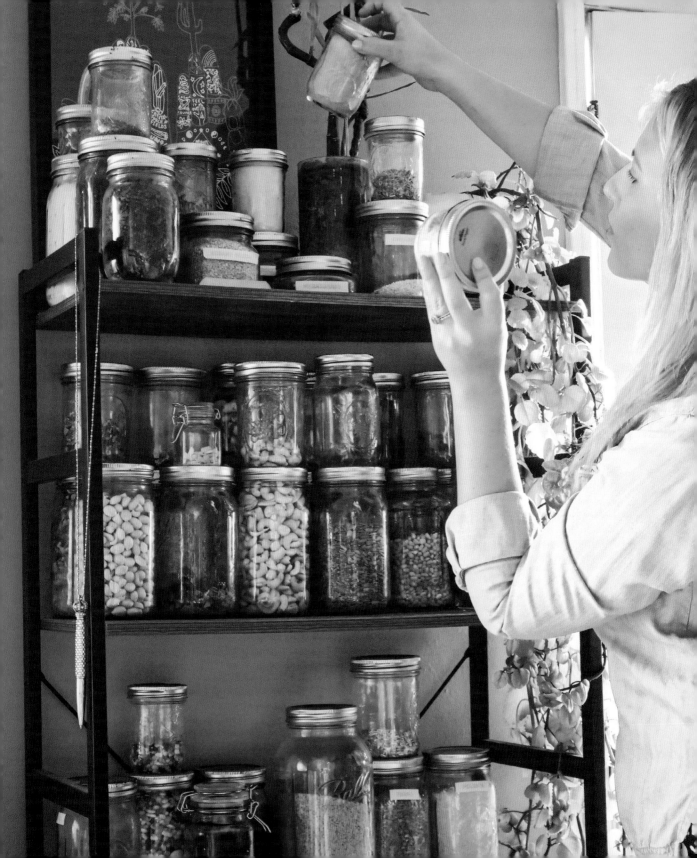

CORE CONCEPTS AND
Ingredients

The main goal for eating a plant-based diet goes beyond eating a delicious meal or two out of this cookbook, although that is definitely going to happen. The bigger picture involves allowing this book to be a tool to help you feel like a true badass in your own kitchen, to help you walk into your home with groceries knowing exactly how you'll use those ingredients to make some magic. It's a process that doesn't happen overnight, but little by little, day after day, you'll start to grow as a cook. Things become less stressful, and eventually, recipes will become more of a guideline than a rule. And I will guide you every step of the way.

If you're a seasoned pro but are new to plant-based cooking, there is still a learning curve. The recipes in this book are designed to take you through many cooking techniques that you can expand on beyond the pages of this cookbook. I use classic techniques with a whole-food, plant-based framework. This chapter can be used as part of your tool belt. The best advice I can give is to dive right in, have patience with yourself and—like you do in life—use every failure as an opportunity to learn.

MIS EN PLACE

Simply translated from French, mis en place means "everything in its place." To have your mis en place is to have all your ingredients ready to go before you start cooking. The recipes written in these pages all start by showing you The Goods, including how to prepare the ingredients if needed, before you

continue on to The Method. This seemingly minor detail is actually a key concept to finding flow in your kitchen. If you prep all your ingredients first—if you chop, dice and mince—your entire cooking experience will be smoother. It'll also give you a chance to practice your knife skills without the stress of something burning behind you.

BUILDING FLAVOR

This is where I see so many people and chefs drop the ball when it comes to plant-based cuisine. This style of eating and cooking is no longer accepted as an afterthought and should be viewed the same way we view any other type of cuisine in terms of flavor. Don't be afraid to try new things: Use spices, find new ways to achieve creaminess, play with acidity and use the best-quality ingredients you can.

When building flavor, we're looking at six pillars: (1) sweetness, (2) saltiness, (3) sourness or acidity, (4) spiciness, (5) fattiness and (6) umami. We all have different preferences, so when you are making your meals, think of these six pillars when you're figuring out how to balance flavors and build depth. If it's too salty or spicy, you may need to add some sweetness or fattiness. If it's too bland, you probably need to add a little acidity—I love lemons and limes, as they brighten things up. If it's too sour, use some fattiness or spiciness to mellow out the flavor. These recipes have all been perfectly balanced so that you can sit back, relax and let the recipes do the work. While you're cooking, taste as you go—this way, you can see how the flavor develops as the recipe cooks!

Flavor from whole-food sources isn't just about lighting up our pleasure centers; it's also a perfect excuse to infuse more nutrients and healing properties into our food. Spices and citrus are powerhouses for our overall health, and using them without hesitation is key! My final tip, as you'll see in many of the recipes, is to season the food with salt lightly as you go. Doing so will help bring out the natural flavors in the ingredients and assist with the cooking process. Flavor comes in many forms and is going to be your passport to joy while cooking and eating in an entirely new way.

INTUITIVE EATING AND COOKING

Intuitive eating is essentially listening to your body, practicing self-care through what you eat and ditching the idea of counting calories. The first step is to pay more attention to what's in your food and how you feel after eating it. At first, it might feel overwhelming and slightly obsessive, but eventually you'll learn what foods and brands make you feel great and which don't. This also isn't about obsessing or creating disordered eating around plant food; it's about having strong ethics and a baseline regarding what you will and will not put into your body. That is where the abundant mindset comes in! I have never felt so abundant with food as I do on a plant-based diet. I don't stress about calories, I eat whenever I'm hungry and I let inspiration guide me.

We can learn to do the same with cooking. Cooking intuitively could be as simple as seasoning something when it feels right or adding an extra ingredient to a recipe that you love. It could also be taking one element of a recipe and adding it to another, like using the hibiscus meat on page 73 as the filling for the flautas on page 70. Intuitive cooking is about letting recipes become guidelines rather than rules. It's about letting your sense of smell or taste help you decide when something is done cooking rather than relying strictly on a timer. Most importantly, intuitive cooking is about letting inspiration and exploration be your guides.

COOKING WITH OIL

There are many controversial ideas around whether to cook with oil. Without going too in-depth on this topic, my take on the matter is that moderation and quality are key when cooking with oil. For the sake of simplicity, most recipes in this book use a small amount of high-quality organic extra virgin olive oil. On occasion, you will see coconut oil and sesame oil for flavor or as a replacement for dairy in a baked dish. If at any point you want to substitute olive oil with avocado oil or grapeseed oil, go for it! If you want to experiment with oil-free cooking or need to eliminate oils for heart health, just use a few tablespoons (15–30 ml) of veggie broth to sauté ingredients. You can also replace oil or butter in baked goods with a nut or sunflower seed butter.

I love a good drizzle of olive oil on a salad or a little coconut oil in a stir-fry. With that said, it's important to be careful about deep-fried foods, processed foods with added oils and using oil in excess. My hope is that this bit of info and guidance will help you stay flexible and able to fully enjoy the recipes within this book, oil-free or not!

SOAKING NUTS AND SEEDS

Soaking nuts and seeds, such as cashews and sesame seeds, overnight in filtered water before cooking with them is a simple trick to aid in digestion and create deliciously creamy sauces. Talk about a win-win. This process can also be referred to as sprouting. If you forget to soak your nuts and seeds ahead of time, just pour almost-boiling water over them fifteen minutes before cooking them to speed up this process.

DAIRY ALTERNATIVES

Vegan Cheese

One of the biggest breakthroughs for me on my vegan journey was learning how to make my own cheese. Cheese was the number one reason why I resisted this lifestyle for so long. I practically lived on Gruyère and Brie cheeses in my early culinary days. Cheese seemed impossible to give up. I know that at first it can seem overwhelming to give up dairy-based cheese and even make your own cheeses. But in actuality, it's quite simple and so delicious! I show you how to make a few of my favorites in the chapter entitled "The Essentials" (page 157), and I also provide a cheese recipe for the Chicago-Style Classic Deep-Dish Pizza (page 51). With that said, I encourage you to take advantage of the many store-bought vegan cheeses when first transitioning to a plant-based diet. Since we're aiming for a whole-food, plant-based diet with this book, these store-bought options would ideally be a small percentage of our weeky food intake—nonetheless, I still love a good splurge once in a while! My favorite brands are Miyoko's, Violife, Kite Hill, Treeline and Parmela Creamery.

Plant Milks

Switching from animal-based to plant-based milk is one of the easiest ways to start making the transition to a plant-based diet. Since we all have different preferences, it may take a few tries for you to land on the type of milk you like. I prefer to make my own milk, and I will show you how to easily do so in this book (page 162). You can buy various types of plant milk from the store, like oat milk, almond milk, cashew milk and hemp milk. Be sure to scan the ingredients before purchasing plant milks—look for minimal ingredients and sugar, keeping in mind that unsweetened varieties are best for cooking. You can use these milks in any recipe that calls for milk, as they work same!

Coconut Milk and Coconut Cream

High-quality coconut milk is a staple ingredient in my kitchen. It's the perfect substitute for heavy cream. When shopping for coconut milk, make sure to read the ingredients. Avoid any coconut milk with preservatives, artificial coconut flavoring, added sugar, added coconut water and ingredients you can't pronounce! This will ensure you're getting a smooth and mild coconut milk, perfect for many savory recipes like curries, mashed potatoes, gravies, soups and cheeses.

Compared to coconut milk, coconut cream has much more fat, it has a more prevalent coconut flavor, it is thicker and richer and it is ideal for baking. I recommend buying coconut milk and coconut cream in cans rather than cartons, as the canned kind has a more consistent quality with minimal ingredients.

BREAKING UP WITH EGGS

This was one of the hardest culinary breakups I went through, as eggs were a staple for me. While eggs are a solid source of protein, they are also packed with cholesterol and fat. In addition, the egg industry is not a friendly industry to chickens or our environment. The good news is that there are a ton of whole-food, high-protein egg replacements that can help you scratch that egg itch or assist you in baking. For breakfast eggs, I will show you how to make a tofu scramble in my recipe for Chilaquiles (page 77) and fried eggs from mung beans in The Ultimate Breakfast Sando (page 119). For baking, just replace 1 egg with 1 banana or ½ cup (130 g) of applesauce. You can also replace a chicken egg with a chia or flax egg, which is made up of ground chia or flax seeds and water. Use this equation: 1 tablespoon (6 g) of ground chia or flax seeds combined with 2½ tablespoons (37 ml) of water equals 1 egg. The key is to slowly start replacing your eggs with alternatives. You'll be surprised at how amazing you feel without them!

Chia and Flax

These are super seeds! Chia and flax are both excellent sources of omega-3, omega-6 and protein. Studies show that the healthiest and most effective way to get a good balance of omega-3 and omega-6 is by consuming them in a whole-food, plant-based form instead of from the popular fish oil supplements or from animal-based foods. Add 1 tablespoon (10 g) of either seed to your smoothie in the morning— you'll be happy you did! Look for them in powdered form, which is ideal for egg replacement (see the preceding section). If you can't find ground flax or chia, place ½ cup (80 g) of whole flax or chia seeds in a dry blender and blend them on high until they turn into a powder.

Black Salt

Black salt, also known as kala namak, is a volcanic rock salt that adds a sulfur-like flavor to any dish. Its primary use in my kitchen is to give that eggy flavor to dishes, but I also love it as a finishing salt. You can find it at your local health-food store or online.

JACKFRUIT

Jackfruit has risen in popularity in the vegan scene over the past few years, and it is crazy cool how mainstream it's become. Jackfruit is a large tropical fruit that originated in India and is in the same family as figs and mulberries. Jackfruit is amazing because when it is unripe, the bulbs make for a perfect, low-sugar meat substitute in recipes. When it's ripe, the jackfruit is delicious in smoothies. Tropical jackfruit is becoming more and more available at local grocery stores—look for canned, unripened jackfruit in brine—which makes your venture into plant-based foods that much easier.

BAKING

Spelt versus Refined Wheat

Spelt is one of my favorite discoveries in the plant world. As a result of my own chronic health issues, for a long time I believed that gluten was to be feared. I noticed a lot of my endometriosis symptoms would flare up anytime I consumed products containing gluten. In reality, there are many whole grains that contain gluten, which proves that not all gluten products are created equal. Gluten is a binding protein often found in grains like wheat, farro, barley, rye and spelt.

If you have a sensitivity to gluten and you do not have celiac disease, there is a chance that you are actually reacting to refined wheat products rather than gluten as a whole. In most Western countries, wheat causes millions of people digestive issues and inflammatory reactions that have nothing to do with celiac disease. This has everything to do the glyphosate sprayed on the wheat crop and the fact that wheat in America is genetically modified, highly processed and, in lots of cases, bleached. It's a recipe for disaster.

The good news? Spelt! Spelt is an amazing whole grain that's delicious and packed with nutrients like fiber, iron, magnesium and zinc, while being lower in gluten than your typical wheat. Spelt is less processed and not genetically modified, making it an almost untouched whole and ancient grain. Spelt is used throughout these pages to show you how truly versatile this grain is. I highly recommend you give spelt a try if you haven't yet. Although it is not gluten-free, it completely changed the game for me and my inflammation—I feel amazing after I eat it rather than bloated and symptomatic. It bakes like white flour but with much more flavor, which can allow for the most delicious and satisfying loaf of bread (page 178). Try spelt next time you need a replacement for white flour.

Gluten Free

Other than the recipes where I use spelt flour, all of the other recipes in this book are gluten-free. I love brown rice pasta for simplicity and added protein, and cassava flour as an amazing starchy flour substitute. You can be sure, no matter what your food allergies are, you will find what you're looking for in this book!

Cacao versus Cocoa

I admit that I am a total chocoholic. I was first introduced to cacao when I took part in cacao ceremonies while hosting retreats. I was amazed at how euphoric cacao can make you feel. The difference between the two is that the popular cocoa is processed at a much higher temperature than cacao and is often packaged with excess sugar and powdered dairy products. Cacao, on the other hand, is often fair-trade, more sustainable and fermented instead of roasted, which helps maintain the plant's high level of antioxidants and will give you that amazing feeling of euphoria. It is slightly more expensive but worth every penny!

Making It Sweet

Alternative, unrefined sweeteners can absolutely change the game for your cooking skills and the way you build flavor. They can also help with reducing sugar intake and avoiding refined sugars completely. I'm not talking about artificial sweeteners, as studies show those sweeteners can actually cause major health problems. I'm talking about good old-fashioned maple syrup, date syrup, agave nectar or coconut sugar! These four are my go-tos when I need an alternative to refined white or brown sugars or corn syrup. They also can play a crucial role in balancing flavors in savory dishes and can be used as replacements for each other in most baked goods. Date syrup and coconut sugar are made directly from plants and are low on the glycemic index. This means that they won't spike your blood sugar as much and can be used in moderation without the worry!

TAPIOCA FLOUR, ARROWROOT POWDER AND CORNSTARCH

These are the three amigos. They all work the same and can be used interchangeably in every single recipe in this book. I prefer tapioca flour for sweet dishes, but other than that caveat, they all go hand in hand. Accessibility and availability make up one of my core beliefs as a chef. No matter where you live, if you have a stocked pantry with flexible ingredients like these, you can make most if not all of the recipes in this book.

SEASONINGS

Nutritional Yeast

You'll see this ingredient often in plant-based cheesy recipes. It is a deactivated yeast that can be found in the spices, baking or condiment section of most grocery stores. It will give your recipes a cheesy flavor while also adding a boost of nutrients like B vitamins—including B12—iron and zinc. Make sure to buy unfortified nutritional yeast when you can, as the fortified variety has unnecessarily added synthetic vitamins and minerals, which are harder for your body to digest. You can use nutritional yeast in cheese recipes, on pasta, in soups and on salads!

Coconut Aminos and Liquid Aminos

Both of these ingredients are epic soy sauce alternatives. I prefer them to soy sauce and tamari because they have a fraction of the sodium. This journey is not just about going vegan—it's about finding heart-healthy alternatives as well. Liquid aminos are made from soybeans and taste like a lighter version of tamari, which is a gluten-free soy sauce. Coconut aminos are made from fermenting the sap of the coconut blossom and have a slightly sweet and less salty flavor than liquid aminos. Both of these are incredibly important staples to have in your kitchen. They assist big-time with building low-sodium flavor profiles and help when you are caramelizing goods in the kitchen.

Miso Paste

Miso paste is one of my go-to ingredients for building flavor! It is made of fermented soybeans or garbanzo beans—for those of you who are sensitive to soy—and has a sweet and salty umami flavor. It is a necessary and affordable staple to have in your fridge at all times, as it has a long shelf life. Miso adds great depth to salad dressings, soups, curries and vegan cheeses! You can find it near wherever you get your tofu in the store. For the recipes in this book, I prefer white miso or garbanzo bean miso. Make sure to look for non-GMO and organic miso when possible.

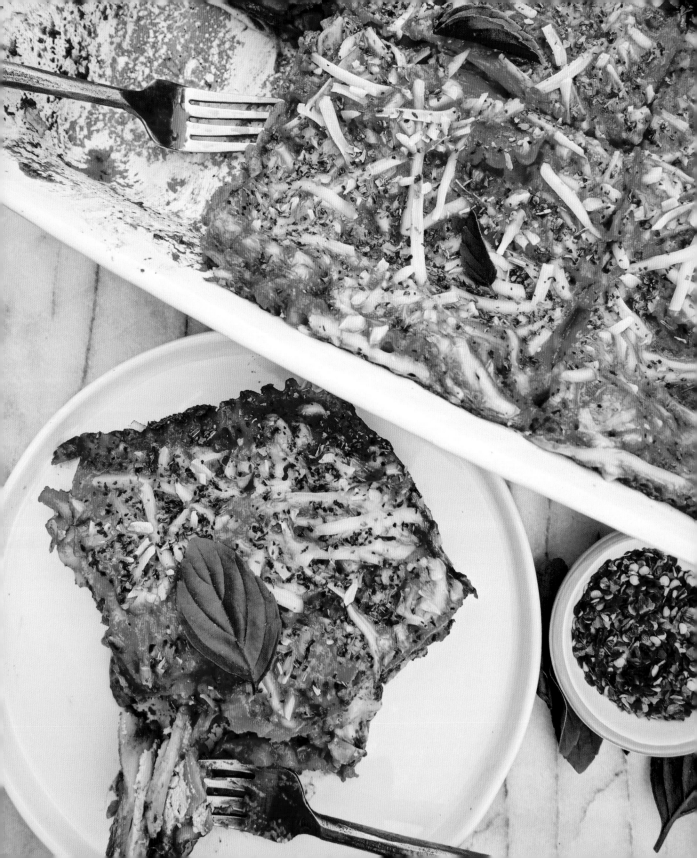

GUILT-FREE *Comfort Food*

This entire chapter is focused on the idea that you truly can have what you want and what you need. There is a common misconception people often have when switching to a plant-focused diet: You'll be giving up your favorite soul foods. I'm talkin' about those foods that make you feel all fuzzy and warm inside. Those foods that bring you nostalgia about your grandmother, a childhood tradition, a time when you stayed home from school sick in bed or those many nights during college when you were too stressed to function.

These are the foods that fuel our souls but rarely do justice for our bodies. Ingredients like heavy cream, butter, refined sugar, refined pastas, bacon fat, white flour, ground beef, cheese and pork are all ingredients that are consumed the most in developed countries and are also the foods that contribute the most to heart disease, diabetes, obesity and cancer—just to name a few. The good news? There are delicious replacements in the plant world for all of these things, which can not only bring you back to your roots but can also heal your body at the same time.

There is always much to be said about and learned from the way our elders did things in the kitchen. It was about love, culture and availability. It was about the idea that you could truly taste love in the food they cooked and the fact that your grandmother was always right, especially when she was cooking.

This chapter pays homage to all of the grandmothers, mothers and other caregivers out there who taught us how to feed our souls in the first place. Everything we ate when we were children has been imprinted on our souls somewhere. As we age, we continue to be imprinted with and reminded of these delicious food-driven memories. These memories drive our choices every day, with every meal we eat, and in a way drive the way we cook as well.

We'll swap out heavy cream for cauliflower and cashews in classic Spaghetti Alfredo (page 16). We'll replace ground beef with mushrooms for all the protein, iron and flavor of a traditional Shepherd's Pie (page 20) and leave behind the saturated fat. I'll show you how to swap pulled pork for jackfruit in my Barbecue Pulled No-Pork Sliders with Slaw and Spelt Buns (page 24), and on page 33 we'll make a plant-based gravy that'll give Betty Crocker a run for her money.

To sum it all up, I will show you how to easily re-create some of your favorite comfort foods and give you the tools you need to find pleasure and comfort in plant-based cuisine.

SPAGHETTI ALFREDO

Traditionally, Alfredo sauce and others like it are packed to the brim with clarified butter, heavy cream, flour and salt. I swear these sauces are where the term food coma comes from! This twist on Alfredo will fulfill all of your creamy pasta dreams without the need for a long nap on the couch afterward. A few key ingredients make this dish so magical. The miso paste adds a specific salty, umami flavor that perfectly rounds out the sauce. The cauliflower is a sneaky way to add a serving of veggies into your day and helps make this sauce irresistibly fluffy and smooth—this Alfredo is the ideal choice for picky eaters or kiddos. Finally, the nutmeg is a trick I learned from my French culinary schoolbooks, as it gives Alfredo its signature flavor!

THE GOODS

SPAGHETTI ALFREDO

1 (1-lb [454-g]) package brown rice spaghetti

½ small cauliflower, cut into florets

1 cup (150 g) raw cashews, soaked in cool water overnight or in hot water for 15 minutes and drained

1 tbsp (20 g) miso paste

¼ tsp black pepper, plus more as needed

¼ tsp ground nutmeg

½ tsp onion powder

¾ tsp granulated garlic

¼ tsp salt, plus more as needed

1¼ cups (300 ml) unsweetened oat milk

1 tbsp (15 ml) fresh lemon juice

TOPPINGS

Walnut Parm (page 161)
Red pepper flakes
Black pepper
Finely chopped fresh parsley

THE METHOD

To make the spaghetti Alfredo, you'll need two large pots: one for the spaghetti and one for the cauliflower.

Fill the pot for the spaghetti three-fourths of the way with water and add a generous pinch of salt. Cover the pot and bring the water to a boil over medium heat. Add the spaghetti and cook it, uncovered, according to the package's instructions. Strain the spaghetti and rinse it with cold water to stop the cooking process, then set the spaghetti aside.

Meanwhile, fill the pot for the cauliflower with 1 inch (2.5 cm) of water and insert a steamer basket. Add the cauliflower florets to the steamer basket, turn the heat on to medium-low, cover the pot and cook the cauliflower for about 10 minutes. You'll know the cauliflower is done when you can easily pierce it with a fork.

Remove the cauliflower from the steamer basket and transfer it to a blender. Add the soaked cashews, miso paste, black pepper, nutmeg, onion powder, granulated garlic, salt, milk and lemon juice to the blender. Blend the ingredients on high speed for about 2 minutes, until they have a smooth consistency. If your blender is struggling a little, just add a bit more milk and blend until the sauce smooths out.

Transfer the sauce and spaghetti to the pot you cooked the pasta in. Turn the heat on low and cook the spaghetti Alfredo for 1 to 2 minutes to heat it up. Season it with additional salt and black pepper to taste. Serve the spaghetti Alfredo in individual bowls topped with the Walnut Parm, red pepper flakes, black pepper and parsley.

BAI'S TIP: This sauce makes an amazing meal prep. Just make the sauce ahead of time and cook the noodles whenever you're ready to dive in! The sauce lasts for 5 to 6 days in the fridge.

Makes 3 to 4 servings

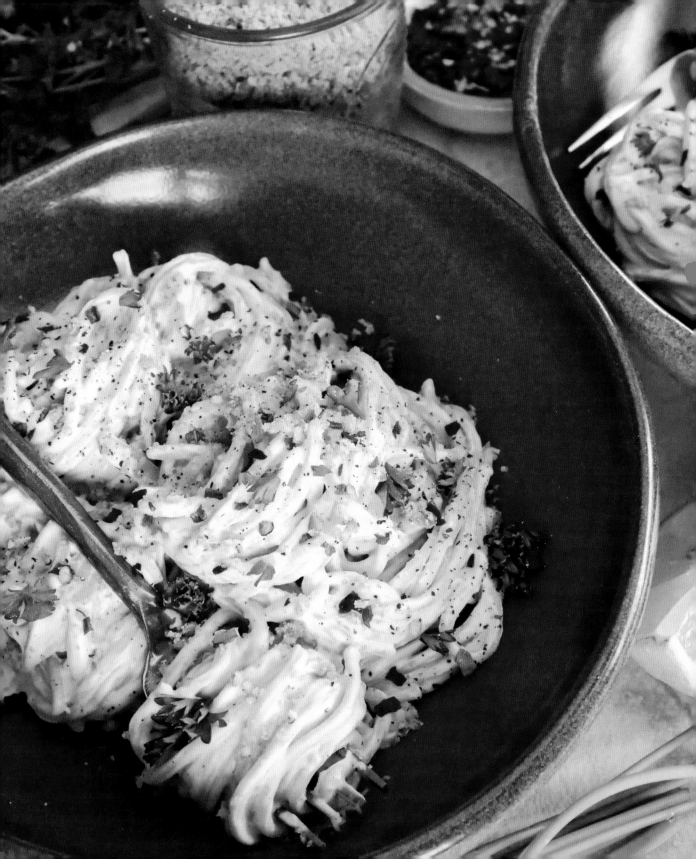

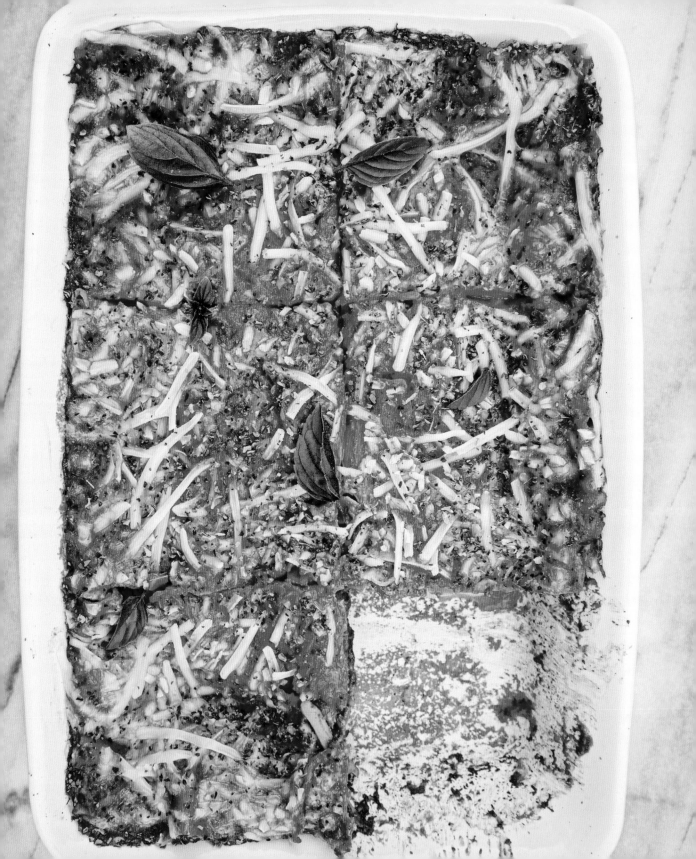

ROASTED RED PEPPER LASAGNA

Satisfying cravings, eating a rainbow of veggies and having a party in your mouth sums up this recipe perfectly. There is so much incredible flavor, creaminess and texture in this lasagna. On the other hand, it's gluten-free and a very sneaky way to get in spinach, beets, mushrooms and plant-based protein. Switching to a new lifestyle or eating in a way that's outside of the "norm" is always better with friends and family, which is why a pan of lasagna like this one fits the bill: great to share, family-friendly, packed with nutrients and completely drool-worthy.

THE GOODS

RED PEPPER SAUCE

3 medium red bell peppers

1 medium beet, peeled and thinly sliced

¾ cup (180 ml) unsweetened plant milk

1 tsp garlic powder

1 tsp onion powder

¾ tsp salt

1 tsp dried basil

¼ tsp black pepper

PESTO

1 large bunch fresh basil, destemmed

2 cups (60 g) baby spinach

3 cloves garlic, peeled

3 tbsp (45 ml) fresh lemon juice

1 tsp black pepper

1 tsp salt

3 tbsp (45 ml) olive oil

2 tbsp (30 ml) water

LASAGNA

2 (1-lb [454-g]) packages brown rice lasagna noodles

1 tbsp (15 ml) olive oil

2½ cups (200 g) thinly sliced cremini mushrooms

¼ tsp salt

1½ cups (410 g) Tofu Ricotta or Almond Ricotta (page 165), divided

1 cup (110 g) shredded vegan mozzarella cheese, divided

1 tsp red pepper flakes

THE METHOD

Preheat your oven to 400°F (204°C). Place the bell peppers and beet on a medium baking sheet. Cook for 25 to 30 minutes until the beet is fork-tender and the bell peppers are blackened and soft.

Meanwhile, make the pesto. In a blender, combine the basil, spinach, garlic, lemon juice, black pepper, salt, oil and water. Blend until the pesto is smooth. Transfer to a bowl and set aside.

Cook the noodles in a 7-quart (7-L) pot according to the package's instructions. Rinse them with cold water, separate them from one another and set them aside. To prepare the mushrooms, heat the oil in a small sauté pan over medium-high heat. Add the mushrooms and salt and sauté for about 5 minutes, until the mushrooms start to brown. Set aside.

Once the peppers are cool enough to handle, peel as much of the thin skins away as you can and remove the tops and seeds. In your blender, combine the bell peppers, beet, milk, garlic powder, onion powder, salt, dried basil and black pepper. Blend until the mixture is super smooth and creamy.

Grab a 9 x 13–inch (23 x 33–cm) baking pan and pour about ½ cup (120 ml) of red pepper sauce on the bottom, making sure to cover the entire surface of the bottom. Place 4 or 5 lasagna noodles on top of the sauce. Spread ¾ cup (205 g) of the Tofu Ricotta on the noodles. Top with more sauce, then more noodles. For the next layer, pour all of the pesto on the noodles, then add the mushrooms and ½ cup (55 g) of the vegan mozzarella cheese. Top this layer with more noodles, then more sauce. Finally, spread the remaining ¾ cup (205 g) of the Tofu Ricotta across the sauce. Add another layer of noodles and the rest of the sauce. Finish with the remaining ½ cup (55 g) of mozzarella and red pepper flakes.

Cover the lasagna with aluminum foil or an ovenproof lid and bake it for 30 minutes. Uncover and bake it for 20 more minutes, until the sauce is bubbling and the edges are crispy. Let it cool for 10 to 15 minutes and serve.

Makes 6 servings

SHEPHERD'S PIE

Growing up as a '90s kid, how I remember shepherd's pie is a testament to how I remember my childhood as a whole. My mom always served it with whatever chicken and potatoes we had left over, with a whole heap of Cheddar cheese melted on the top. I wanted to bring those weeknight comfort memories to our modern lives and our health goals. Happiness can be as simple as shepherd's pie and a loved one to share it with. Simple, oh so satisfying and good for you too.

THE GOODS

2½ lb (1.1 kg) yellow potatoes, diced into medium pieces

8 cloves garlic, thinly sliced, divided

3 tsp (18 g) salt, divided, plus more as needed

1 tsp black pepper, divided, plus more as needed

3 tbsp (45 ml) melted Not Your Mama's Salted Butter (page 158) or store-bought vegan butter

1 cup (240 ml) unsweetened plant milk

1 tbsp (15 ml) olive oil

½ medium red onion, thinly sliced

1 large carrot, finely chopped

2 medium ribs celery, finely chopped

2 heaping tbsp (50 g) tomato paste

⅔ cup (160 ml) red wine

3 cups (240 g) thinly sliced cremini mushrooms

2 cups (480 ml) Immune-Boosting Veggie Broth (page 170)

1 cup (130g) fresh or frozen corn kernels

¼ cup (60 ml) water

2 tbsp (19 g) cornstarch

3 large leaves rainbow chard, destemmed and sliced

Walnut Parm (page 161), as needed

Dried herb blend, for garnish (optional)

THE METHOD

Preheat the oven to 350°F (177°C). Then fill a 5- to 7-quart (5- to 7-L) pot halfway with water. Add the potatoes, 5 cloves of the garlic, 1 teaspoon of the salt and ½ teaspoon of the black pepper. Bring the water to a boil over high heat. Reduce the heat a little and cook for about 10 minutes, or until the potatoes are fork-tender.

Drain the potatoes and garlic and transfer to a stand mixer or a large bowl. Add the butter and milk, then mix or use a potato masher to mash them until smooth and creamy. Taste it, and add additional salt and black pepper—I like my potatoes a little salty! Set aside.

Next, heat the oil in a large sauté pan over medium heat. Toss in the onion and a pinch of salt. Cook for 2 to 3 minutes, until softened. Add the carrot, celery, 1 teaspoon of the salt and the remaining ½ teaspoon black pepper and cook the mixture for 1 minute. Toss in the remaining 3 cloves of garlic and the tomato paste and mix the ingredients until everything is covered in the tomato paste. If the mixture is starting to burn on the bottom, that's what the wine is for: Pour in the wine and cook the vegetables for 3 to 5 minutes, until the liquid until has evaporated, then add the mushrooms. Cook the mushrooms for 2 to 3 minutes, until they have reduced in size, then add the broth and corn. Stir the mixture, cover, reduce the heat to medium-low and cook for 3 to 5 more minutes.

Meanwhile, combine the water and cornstarch in a small bowl to create a slurry. Uncover the sauté pan, add the slurry and mix until the slurry is fully dissolved. Finally, add the chard, cook for 1 minute, taste and adjust the saltiness as needed. Cover the pan and remove it from the heat.

Grab a large cast-iron skillet or a 9 x 11–inch (23 x 28–cm) baking dish and pour in the gravy-veggie mixture. Scoop your mashed potatoes on top, spreading them evenly. Top with a generous amount of the Walnut Parm. Bake it for 15 minutes, until the gravy is bubbling and the potatoes are starting to brown. Season the shepherd's pie with the remaining 1 teaspoon of salt. Serve the shepherd's pie piping hot in bowls with a sprinkling of dried herbs if desired.

Makes 4 servings

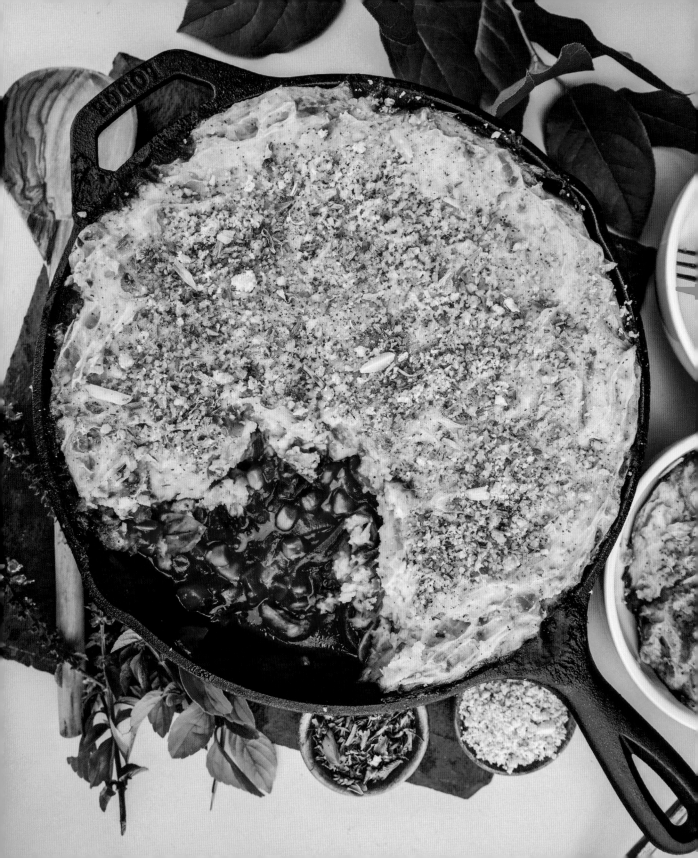

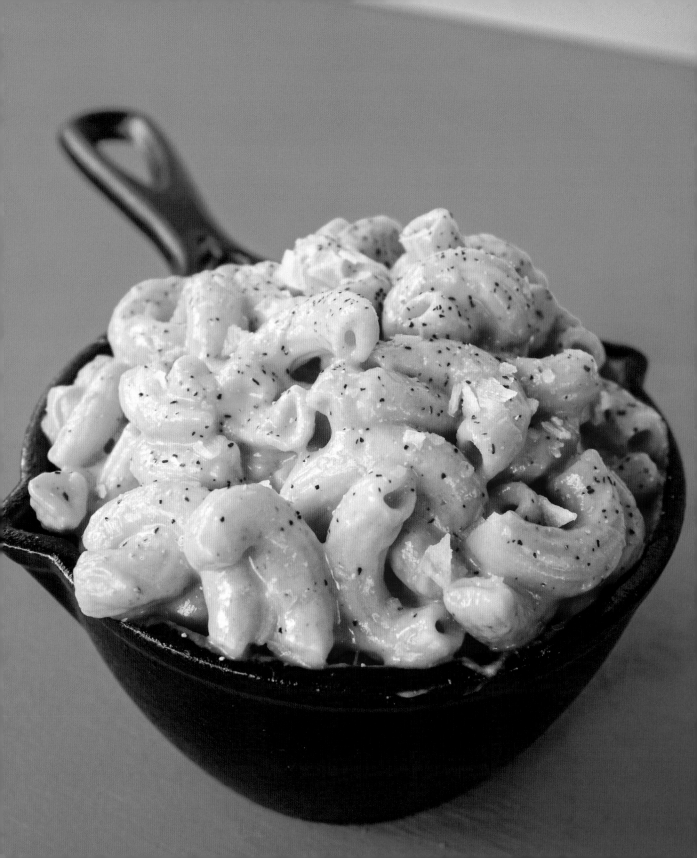

MAC 'N' CHEESY GOODNESS

Cheesy cravings activated by a dish made entirely of veggies? Oh, you better believe it. This recipe is so damn delicious and hits every single spot. Traditional mac and cheese has been ruined by processed powders in boxes and a dairy industry that is a nightmare for the environment, the animals who are born into the industry and our bodies. It's a depressing thought that a dish that brought us so much joy as children—and adults—actually isn't as wholesome and wonderful as we were led to believe. To avoid depressing you too much, I will say with full confidence that this recipe has the potential to change your life and the way you experience cravings. Kids and adults alike love this gluten-free recipe, as it's perfect for a quick and healthy lunch in the middle of a school day or for a lunch gathering with friends. It whips up almost as fast as the boxed version—you'll be wondering why you didn't make the switch sooner!

THE GOODS

2 small yellow potatoes, coarsely chopped

2 large carrots, coarsely chopped

1 medium yellow onion, coarsely chopped

3 cloves garlic, peeled

½ cup (75 g) raw cashews

2 tsp (12 g) salt, divided, plus more as needed

1 lb (454 g) brown rice elbow pasta

1 cup (240 ml) unsweetened plant milk

1 tbsp (20 g) miso paste

1 tbsp (5 g) nutritional yeast

1 tsp ground turmeric

½ tsp black pepper, plus more as needed

THE METHOD

Fill a large saucepan halfway with water. Add the potatoes, carrots, onion, garlic, cashews and 1 teaspoon of the salt. Bring the water to a boil over high heat. Reduce the heat to medium and cook the veggies for 10 minutes, or until the potatoes and carrots are fork-tender.

While the veggies are cooking, cook your pasta according to the package's instructions. Drain the pasta and rinse it with cold water. This step is key for brown rice pasta. Set the pasta aside in the pot you cooked it in.

Drain the water from your veggies and transfer them to a blender. Add the remaining 1 teaspoon of salt, milk, miso paste, nutritional yeast, turmeric and black pepper. Blend the ingredients on medium speed for about 1 minute, until they are smooth. Pour the cheesy goodness over the pasta. Turn the heat to low, mix the sauce and pasta well and heat the pasta up. Divide the pasta between two or three serving bowls. Top each serving with additional black pepper and salt to taste.

Makes 2 to 3 servings

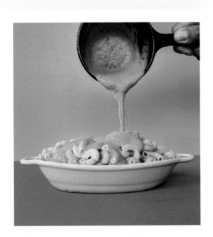

BARBECUE PULLED NO-PORK SLIDERS WITH SLAW AND SPELT BUNS

Barbecued meat is an American tradition that a lot of people don't take lightly. This recipe is no exception, except we've got the pigs in mind and are using jackfruit instead! Jackfruit works as a delicious meat replacement and happens to be high in fiber. This fact puts this recipe high on our list for gut health. It's totally possible to avoid refined carbs, refined sugars and processed meats and still get the "real thing." You've got 30-minute spelt buns, a sweet and tangy barbecue sauce and a simple slaw locked and loaded to make your next backyard shindig one for the books.

THE GOODS

SPELT BUNS

2 tbsp (18 g) active dry yeast

¼ cup (40 g) coconut sugar or sweetener of choice

1 cup (240 ml) water, warmed to about 105°F (41°C)

⅓ cup (80 ml) olive oil

1 tbsp (6 g) ground chia seeds combined with 3 tbsp (45 ml) water

½ tsp salt

2¾ to 3 cups (440 to 480 g) spelt flour

Melted Not Your Mama's Salted Butter (page 158) or store-bought vegan butter, as needed

1 tbsp (9 g) black or white sesame seeds

BARBECUE JACKFRUIT

½ cup (200 g) tomato paste

¼ cup (60 ml) water

2 tbsp (30 ml) molasses

1 tbsp (15 ml) apple cider vinegar

2 tbsp (30 ml) pure maple syrup

1 tbsp (15 ml) plus 1 tsp olive oil, divided

½ tsp mustard powder

½ tsp garlic powder

½ tsp onion powder

½ tsp black pepper

1 tsp ground cumin

1 tsp paprika

1 tsp salt, plus more as needed

THE METHOD

Start by making your buns so they have time to rise while you make the rest of the meal. Preheat the oven to 475°F (246°C). Line a large baking sheet with parchment paper.

In a large bowl, combine the yeast, sugar and water. Let the mixture sit for about 5 minutes to give the yeast a chance to bloom. It'll be ready when you see a layer of foam on the top of the water.

Next, add the oil and the chia mixture. Mix the ingredients well with a fork, add the salt and then slowly add the flour 1 cup (160 g) at a time. Mix the dough with a fork at first; when it starts to come together, you can switch to kneading it with your hands. Stop adding the flour when the dough is no longer wet but is still a little sticky and is kneading easily. Knead the dough five to seven times, until the dough springs back when you touch it. Divide the dough into 10 balls. You may need to knead each bun once or twice to get the perfect shape. Place each bun on the prepared baking sheet about 2 inches (5 cm) apart. Cover the buns with a dish towel and let them rise on the counter for 20 minutes. Do not let them rise on the stove, as the oven is preheating.

While the buns are rising, make your barbecue jackfruit. In a medium bowl, whisk together the tomato paste, water, molasses, vinegar, maple syrup, 1 tablespoon (15 ml) of the oil, mustard powder, garlic powder, onion powder, black pepper, cumin, paprika and salt. Set the sauce aside.

(continued)

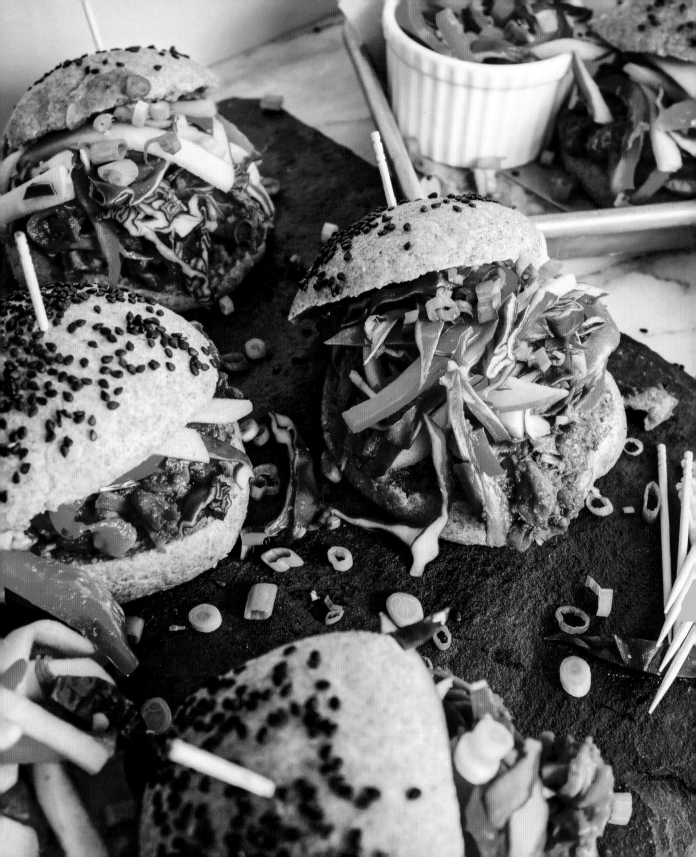

1 small yellow onion, thinly sliced

2 (20-oz [567-g]) cans jackfruit, drained, rinsed and coarsely chopped

SLAW

2 cups (180 g) thinly sliced cabbage

1 large apple, thinly sliced

1 medium red bell pepper, thinly sliced

1 tbsp (15 ml) pure maple syrup

1 tbsp (15 ml) fresh lemon juice

1 tbsp (15 ml) apple cider vinegar

½ tsp salt

Heat the remaining 1 teaspoon of oil in a deep sauté pan over medium-high heat. Add the onion with a pinch of salt. Cook the onion for about 1 minute, then add the jackfruit. Sear the jackfruit and onion for 2 to 3 minutes, giving them a chance to cook together without the sauce. Add the sauce and stir the jackfruit to coat it in the sauce. Turn the heat down to low, cover the sauté pan and cook the jackfruit for about 20 minutes, stirring it about every 5 minutes.

Now that your jackfruit is gettin' sauced, uncover your buns, brush them with the melted butter and sprinkle each with the sesame seeds. Bake them for 10 to 12 minutes—they will start to turn golden brown when they are done. Let them cool on the baking sheet.

While your buns are baking and your jackfruit is doing its thing, make your slaw. Grab a large bowl and combine the cabbage, apple, bell pepper, maple syrup, lemon juice, vinegar and salt. Mix the slaw well, taste it for seasoning and get ready for sliders.

Assemble the sliders by cutting the slightly cooled buns in half, adding the barbecue jackfruit on the bottom half, then adding the slaw on top and topping the sliders with the top half of the bun.

BAI'S TIP: Can't find canned jackfruit? Use garbanzo beans or mushrooms instead! If you can't find ground chia seeds, make your own by blending 1 cup (160 g) of chia seeds in a dry blender until you get a powder. Flaxseed meal is a great replacement also.

Makes 10 sliders

CAULIFLOWER WINGS WITH HOUSE RANCH

I'll be honest: Whenever I've gone to a sporting event, it's been for the food rather than for the sports. Sporting events are the perfect excuse to veg out with a beer or cider and grub down in the company of friends! There's food on the grill, dips, popcorn, cheese fries—but let's be real, the ultimate party food is wings. A dozen chicken wings might sound appealing, but the reality is that one dozen wings contains 60 grams of fat, 480 milligrams of cholesterol and six chickens' lives. Yikes. With that said, you're probably wondering if cauliflower can really do the job—and my answer is a big fat yes! You get that soft interior with a crispy exterior. These wings are baked, not fried, and there are two epic sauces to choose from with a creamy ranch dip to go with both. You can also pair these wings with the barbecue sauce from page 24! To make enough wings to go with both sauces, double the batch of wings. Your friends will love these wings and your heart will thank you for them, but your taste buds will be the real winners in this game.

THE GOODS

WINGS

1 large cauliflower

1 cup (120 g) quinoa flour or brown rice flour

¾ cup (180 ml) unsweetened plant milk

¾ cup (180 ml) water

½ tsp garlic powder

½ tsp salt

½ tsp paprika

HOUSE RANCH

1 cup (150 g) raw cashews, soaked in cool water overnight or in hot water for 15 minutes and drained

½ cup (120 ml) unsweetened plant milk

1 tsp white wine vinegar

½ tsp apple cider vinegar

1 tsp granulated garlic

1 tsp onion powder

1 tsp salt

½ tsp black pepper

¼ cup (12 g) finely chopped fresh dill

THE METHOD

To make the wings, preheat your oven to 400°F (204°C). Line a large baking sheet with parchment paper.

Remove the florets from the cauliflower. Cut them into bite-sized pieces and set them aside. Grab a large bowl and whisk together the flour, milk, water, garlic powder, salt and paprika. Once the ingredients have combined into a smooth batter, dip each cauliflower wing into the batter. Place each coated wing on the prepared baking sheet. Bake the wings for 50 to 60 minutes. During the last 5 minutes of baking time, toss the cauliflower and increase the oven's temperature to broil to get that crispiness we all love. The wings should be golden brown and fork-tender.

While your wings are cooking, you have plenty of time to make your sauces! To make the ranch, combine the cashews, milk, white wine vinegar, apple cider vinegar, granulated garlic, onion powder, salt and black pepper in a high-powered blender. Blend the ingredients until they are smooth. Pour the ranch into a serving bowl and mix in the dill.

(continued)

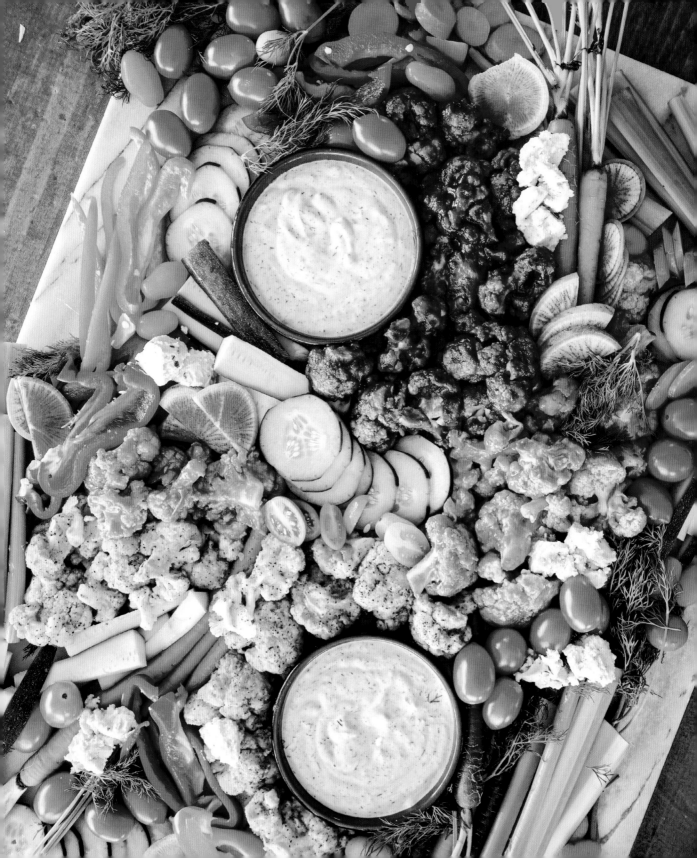

LEMON-PEPPER SAUCE

2 tbsp (30 ml) melted Not Your Mama's Salted Butter (page 158) or store-bought vegan butter

¼ cup (60 ml) fresh lemon juice

½ tsp salt

1 tsp black pepper

MEXI-CALI BUFFALO SAUCE

½ cup (120 ml) melted Not Your Mama's Salted Butter (page 158) or store-bought vegan butter

½ cup (120 ml) Mexican hot sauce (such as Valentina, Tapatío or Cholula® brands)

2 tbsp (30 ml) white wine vinegar

1 tbsp (15 ml) vegan Worcestershire sauce

1 tsp ground coriander

½ tsp garlic powder

¼ tsp salt

To make the lemon-pepper sauce, whisk together the butter, lemon juice, salt and black pepper in a large bowl.

To make the Mexi-Cali Buffalo sauce, whisk together the butter, hot sauce, white wine vinegar, Worcestershire sauce, coriander, garlic powder and salt in a large bowl.

Once your wings are done, toss them in the sauces. Serve the wings with the ranch and devour them immediately.

BAI'S TIP: To make this recipe into a party platter, make the lemon-pepper sauce and the Mexi-Cali Buffalo sauce from this recipe as well as the Barbecue Jackfruit sauce on page 24. Make enough wings for all three sauces. Arrange the wings, along with the ranch for dipping, on a large cutting board or platter with your choice of carrots, bell peppers, Herbed Creamy Feta (page 166), fresh dill, radishes, celery, zucchini and cherry tomatoes.

Makes 2 to 3 servings

BUTTERNUT SQUASH AND SAGE RISOTTO

Risotto has those French and Italian vibes we're all lookin' for on a cozy date night. Soft rice, fresh herbs, creaminess and amazing flavor to match. Don't be intimidated to make risotto plant-based— it's actually quite simple. A slow cook with lots of love makes this dish perfect to serve the people you adore the most. With all the stirring, you'll get the chance to infuse this dish with all your amazing energy. When you pair this risotto with a chenin blanc, there's no point in going out to eat when date night just got elevated to a whole new level!

THE GOODS

1 tbsp (15 g) Not Your Mama's Salted Butter (page 158) or store-bought vegan butter or olive oil

1 large shallot, minced

1 tsp salt, divided

1 small butternut squash, peeled, deseeded and finely diced

3 cloves garlic, thinly sliced

½ tsp black pepper

1 cup (190 g) arborio rice

1 tsp finely chopped fresh sage

3½ cups (840 ml) Immune-Boosting Veggie Broth (page 170), plus more as needed

1 cup (240 ml) unsweetened plant milk

Fresh sage leaves, as needed

Shaved vegan Parmesan cheese, as needed (see Bai's Tips)

THE METHOD

In a large and deep sauté pan over medium-low heat, melt the butter. Add the shallot and ½ teaspoon of the salt. Stir the shallot for about 30 seconds, until it softens and slightly browns. Add the squash, garlic and black pepper. Cook the mixture for 3 to 4 minutes while stirring it to slightly cook the squash. Add the rice and chopped sage next and cook the mixture for about 1 minute while stirring it to lightly toast the rice. Be careful not to walk away, as this step needs your undivided attention.

Next, add the broth ½ cup (120 ml) at a time. Cook the rice, stirring it frequently, for 3 to 5 minutes between each addition of broth, so that the rice can fully absorb the broth. When you add the last ½ cup (120 ml) of broth, add the milk with it and cook the rice until the liquid is fully absorbed. Taste your rice for doneness: If it is still a little chewy, add another ½ cup (120 ml) of broth and cook it until it is tender. Add the remaining ½ teaspoon of salt, adjusting the amount to your taste if needed.

Divide the risotto among two or three bowls and garnish each serving with a few small sage leaves and vegan Parmesan cheese. Fresh sage leaves are super intense, so start with small ones and build up from there.

BAI'S TIPS: If butternut squash and sage are out of season, replace them with 2 cups (140 g) coarsely chopped mushrooms and 1 teaspoon of finely chopped fresh rosemary. So delicious either way!

I like the Violife brand blocks of vegan Parmesan, which shred and shave amazingly well.

Makes 2 to 3 servings

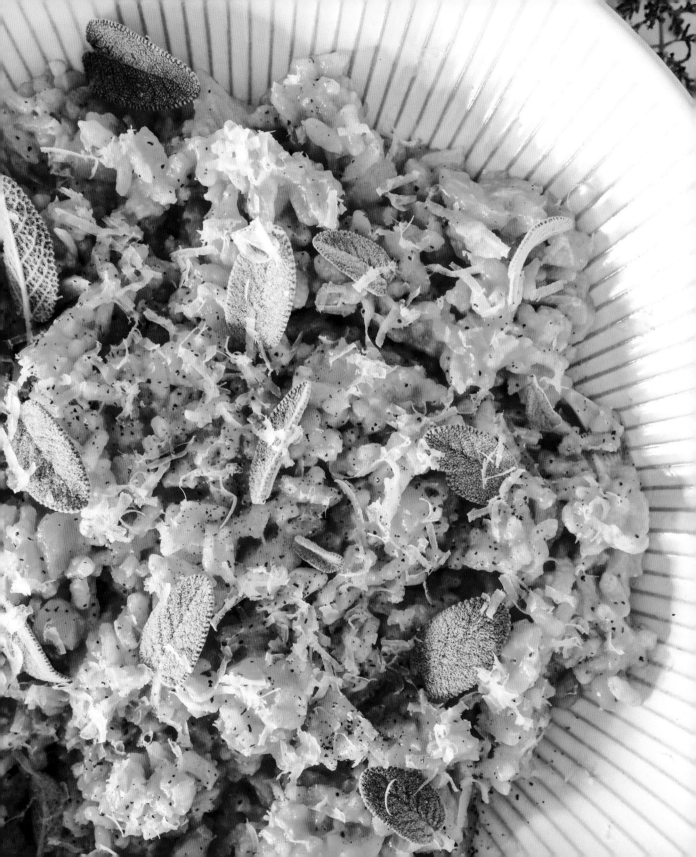

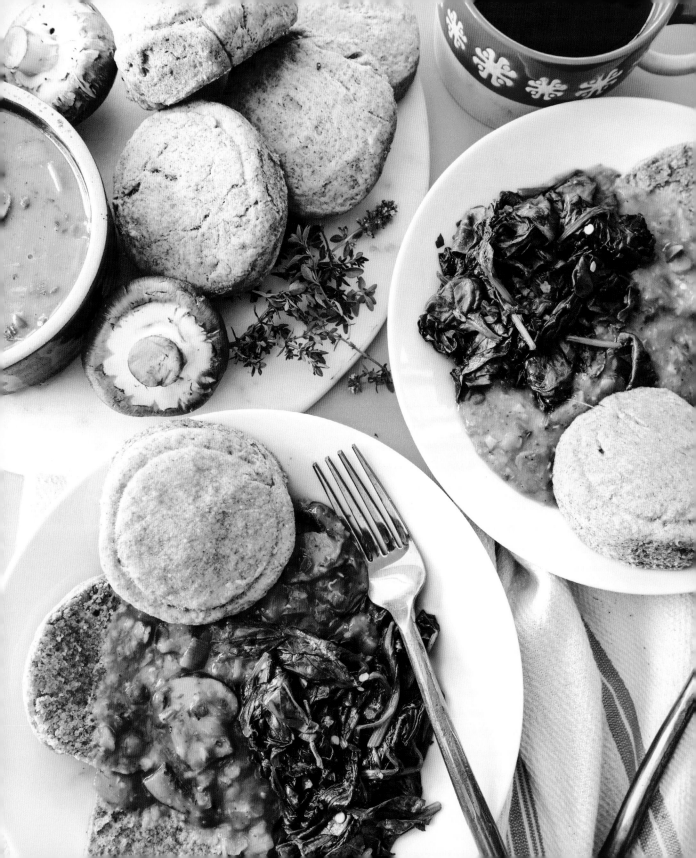

FLAKY, BUTTERY BISCUITS AND MUSHROOM GRAVY

Nothin' says comfort quite like biscuits and gravy. As much as I love this traditional dish, I tend to plan out my naps before diving into a bowl of this much comfort. You can officially let go of the idea that this type of comfort food is designed to make you feel heavy, because I have designed this recipe to make you feel the exact opposite. This entire dish is packed with iron, plant-based proteins, whole grains and healthy fats. I even threw in some sautéed spinach so dark leafy greens could join the party too. Say goodbye to post-biscuit naptime, because this is food for fuel!

THE GOODS

MUSHROOM GRAVY

1 tbsp (15 ml) olive oil

1 medium leek, tops and end removed, thinly sliced

1 small yellow onion, diced

1 tsp salt

2 cloves garlic, minced

1 tbsp (1 g) fresh thyme leaves

½ tsp black pepper

½ cup (120 ml) white wine (optional)

5 cups (400 g) thinly sliced cremini mushrooms

¼ cup (50 g) green lentils, rinsed

4 cups (960 ml) Immune-Boosting Veggie Broth (page 170), divided

1 cup (240 ml) coconut milk

SLURRY

½ cup (120 ml) water

¼ cup (36 g) arrowroot powder

THE METHOD

To make the mushroom gravy, heat the oil in a large sauté pan over medium-high heat. Add the leek, onion and salt. Cook this mixture for 2 to 3 minutes, stirring it frequently with a wooden spoon. Add the garlic, thyme and black pepper. Mix the ingredients together and cook for 1 minute, until the mixture is starting to brown. Add the wine (if using) to deglaze the pan, and cook the mixture for about 2 minutes, until the wine has reduced and there is no liquid left.

Add the mushrooms and cook them for 2 to 3 minutes, until they are starting to brown. Add the lentils and cook them for 30 seconds to slightly toast them.

Next, add 3 cups (720 ml) of the broth. Cover the pan, reduce the heat to low and cook the mixture for 20 minutes. After 20 minutes, you'll notice that most of the liquid has been sucked up by those lentils. Now you'll add the remaining 1 cup (240 ml) of broth and the coconut milk.

Increase the heat to medium. Cook this creamy goodness for 5 minutes. Meanwhile, make the slurry. In a small bowl, mix together the water and arrowroot powder. Add the slurry mixture to the mushrooms and lentils—it will thicken the gravy. Increase the heat to medium-high and cook the gravy for 5 minutes, stirring it frequently. You'll notice your gravy will start to thicken and reach that perfect gravy consistency. Remove the pan from the heat and cover it to keep it warm.

While your gravy is cooking, prepare your biscuits. Preheat your oven to 425°F (218°C). Line a medium baking sheet with parchment paper.

(continued)

BISCUITS

2¼ cups (360 g) spelt flour, plus more as needed

½ tsp salt

1 tbsp (12 g) baking powder

½ tsp baking soda

6 tbsp (90 g) very cold Not Your Mama's Salted Butter (page 158) or store-bought vegan butter (see Bai's Tips), plus more, melted, as needed

¾ cup (180 ml) cold unsweetened plant milk (see Bai's Tips)

SPINACH

1 tbsp (15 ml) olive oil or Immune-Boosting Veggie Broth (page 170)

4 packed cups (400 g) baby spinach

¼ tsp salt

1 tbsp (15 ml) fresh lemon juice

In a large bowl, combine the flour, salt, baking powder and baking soda. Mix the ingredients with a fork until they are well combined. Add the cold butter and cut it into the flour with a pastry cutter or fork. You'll begin to notice pea-sized balls forming—once that happens, stop mixing.

Slowly pour the milk into the flour mixture and mix the two with your fork until they start to form into a ball. You can then knead the dough four or five times with your hands. If it's getting sticky, don't be afraid to dust it with more flour. If it feels a little dry, you can add a splash more of plant milk. It's important not to overmix here, as we still want some pieces of butter in the dough.

Lightly dust a work surface with flour. Press out your buttery dough with your hands on the prepared work surface to create a 1½-inch (4-cm)-thick sheet of dough. Cut out your biscuits with the rim of glass or a Mason jar lid—you should get 8 to 9 dough rounds. Place the dough rounds on the prepared baking sheet, with the edges of the rounds touching, and brush the tops with the melted butter. Bake the biscuits for 12 minutes, just until they are golden brown.

To make the spinach, heat the oil or veggie broth in a small skillet over medium-high heat. Add the spinach, salt and lemon juice and cook the spinach for 2 to 3 minutes, until it cooks down.

Set out four shallow bowls. Place two biscuits in each bowl, then top the biscuits with the gravy and finish it off with your spinach. Enjoy the biscuits and gravy immediately!

BAI'S TIPS: I like to pop the butter in the freezer while I prep the gravy and leave the milk in the fridge until the last minute to make sure they stay extra cold, as temperature is key.

This gravy is a staple in our house and is epic on mashed potatoes! You can also sub the lentils with ground walnuts and half the amount of broth for a faster gravy.

Makes 4 servings

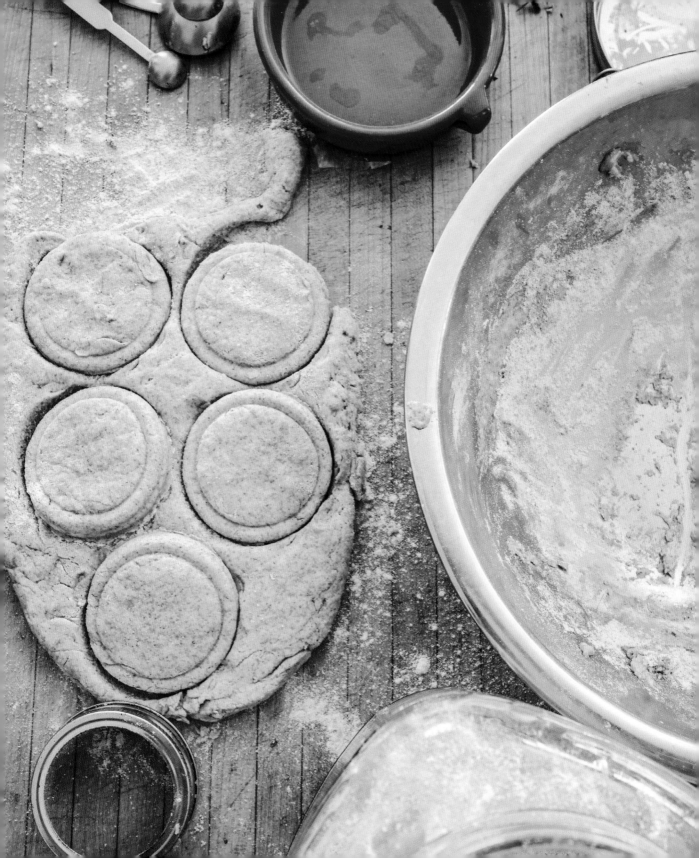

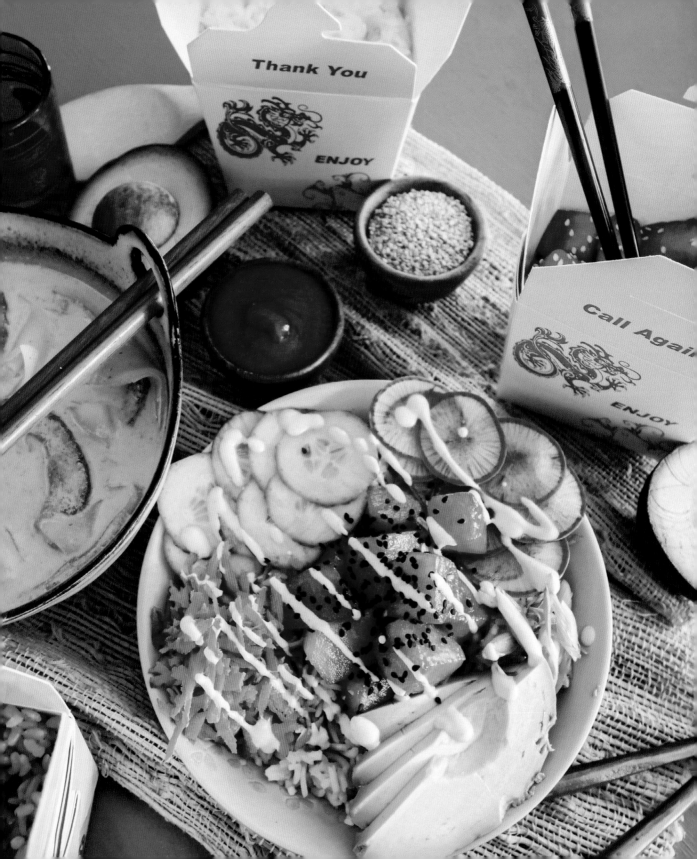

BETTER THAN *Takeout*

Don't get me wrong—I am a huge fan of takeout and an even bigger fan of supporting local restaurants, as they need us more than ever right now. I am also a huge fan of saving money, reducing my sodium intake and knowing exactly what's going into my food. This chapter is not only an ode to our favorite hole-in-the-wall takeout restaurants but it's also an opportunity to grow as a cook and learn how to make things you normally get when you're feeling too lazy to cook.

As a society, we've leaned too hard into the idea that convenience is more important than anything. At first, the drive-through revolutionized the way people ate, but now that same concept is a huge contributor to the ever-growing health crisis we find ourselves in. Nutrients and intention are lost when we eat this way. Profit becomes a bigger factor than ethics, and cutting corners for the margin's sake means that the consumer is the one who suffers. Let's take back our power and feed our bodies, minds and souls before we feed into convenience!

The reality is that we can have our takeout favorites and take care of our bodies. I personally love a good Chinese takeout night or a local pizza delivery. The idea is to supplement some of those days you would normally get that takeout meal with the recipes in this chapter. This is important especially if you suffer from diabetes, high blood pressure, heart disease, obesity, skin problems, high cholesterol or endometriosis, as these issues can be managed much more easily by cooking your favorite takeout meals at home.

Let's jump into the world of homemade takeout together, where food is baked, not fried. Where we use coconut aminos instead of soy sauce and spelt instead of refined bleached flour. These small switches make a huge difference in our long-term health and provide much more flavor than you might think! Cooking with coconut aminos actually changed the way I look at Asian-style food and has helped many people, including my dad, get their blood pressure down by reducing their sodium intake.

After learning to cook your own takeout food, you will be more aware of the food you decide to eat when you do get takeout. You'll start to take more interest in the ingredients and practices of the establishments you support. In actuality, most people have no idea how good they can truly feel—suddenly you'll be so excited to cook your veganized versions from home rather than get takeout!

In this chapter, we'll make a few of my personal takeout favorites. We'll transform the traditional orange chicken (page 49) and learn how to make a green Thai curry, California-style (page 45). We'll cook Indian flavors with ease and make some classics, like Chana Saag and Gluten-Free Garlic Naan (page 41). Pizza is a huge focus in this chapter, and you'll learn to create a crazy delicious deep-dish pizza completely from scratch (page 51). This chapter will open your mind and teach you to build flavors like never before. These recipes are tasty, crave-worthy, nutrient-dense and—believe it or not—better than takeout.

MISO-MUSHROOM RAMEN

Ramen—real ramen—is one of the most magical and delicious soup experiences you can have as a human here on Earth. Authentic Japanese ramen has perfectly balanced umami flavors, noodles to die for and toppings like fried black garlic, chili oil, seaweed, scallions, corn, crispy mushrooms, bok choy . . . I could go on forever. Traditionally, a really good ramen broth has a base of pork and takes hours to make. After making vegan ramen for years now, I'm here to tell you that you can get that umami flavor entirely from plants in under an hour if you have the right ingredients. If you're new to ramen, or if you've been obsessed like I have for a while now, this recipe will become a new staple on your weeknight rotation.

THE GOODS

RAMEN

1 medium acorn squash, thinly sliced and seeds removed

1 (14-oz [397-g]) block firm tofu, drained and lightly pressed (see Bai's Tips on page 133)

1 tbsp (15 ml) toasted sesame oil

1 tbsp (15 ml) coconut aminos

1 tsp granulated garlic

1 tsp pure maple syrup

1 tsp Sriracha

1 (10-oz [283-g]) package ramen noodles

3–4 oz (85–113 g) enoki mushrooms (see Bai's Tips)

Seaweed sheets, crumbled, as needed

BROTH

1 tsp sesame oil

1 medium onion, thinly sliced

1 tsp finely chopped fresh ginger

2 cloves garlic, finely chopped

2 cups (160 g) thinly sliced shiitake mushrooms

¼ cup (80 g) miso paste

1 tsp coconut aminos

1 (14-oz [414-ml]) can light or full-fat coconut milk

5 cups (1.2 L) Immune-Boosting Veggie Broth (page 170)

THE METHOD

To make the ramen, preheat the oven to 400°F (204°C). Line a large baking sheet with parchment paper or a silicone baking mat. Arrange the squash on a baking sheet, then place the block of tofu next to the squash.

In a small Mason jar, combine the sesame oil, coconut aminos, granulated garlic, maple syrup and Sriracha. Mix well, and then pour the mixture over the tofu and the squash. Use your hands to make sure the sauce gets over all of the tofu and squash. Bake for 40 minutes, flipping the tofu halfway through the cooking time, until the squash is fork-tender and the tofu is browned on all sides.

Meanwhile, make the broth. Heat a 5-quart (5-L) pot over medium heat. Add the sesame oil and onion and cook for 2 minutes, stirring frequently. Add the ginger, garlic and shiitake mushrooms. Cook for 1 to 2 minutes, stirring frequently, until the mushrooms have reduced in size a bit. Add the miso paste and coconut aminos. Stir to coat the mushrooms with the miso, and then add your milk and broth. Cover the pot and cook the broth for 15 minutes to allow the flavors to deepen.

Finally, while the broth is cooking, cook your ramen noodles according to the package's instructions, then drain and divide them among three or four soup bowls. Top the noodles with your desired amount of broth and a few pieces of the cooked squash—the skin is edible, and it's up to you if you'd like to peel it off before serving the ramen. Thinly slice your tofu and add two or three slices to each bowl. Finish each serving with 1 ounce (28 g) of the enoki mushrooms, the seaweed and any other toppings you'd like.

BAI'S TIPS: If you have leftovers, make sure to store the noodles separately from the broth or they will get mushy. Look for enoki mushrooms at health-food stores and Asian supermarkets. If you are having trouble finding them, use oyster mushrooms instead.

Makes 3 to 4 servings

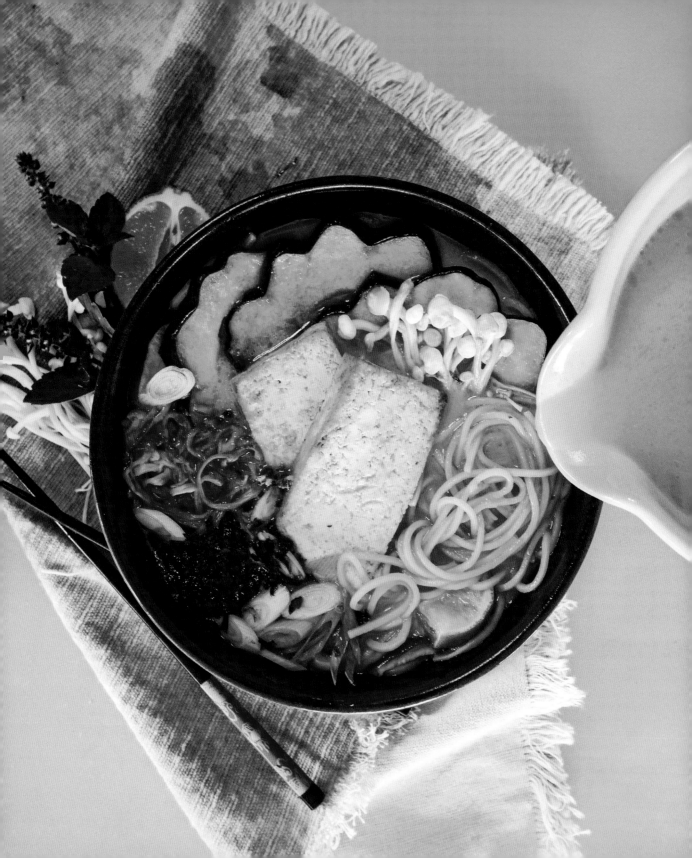

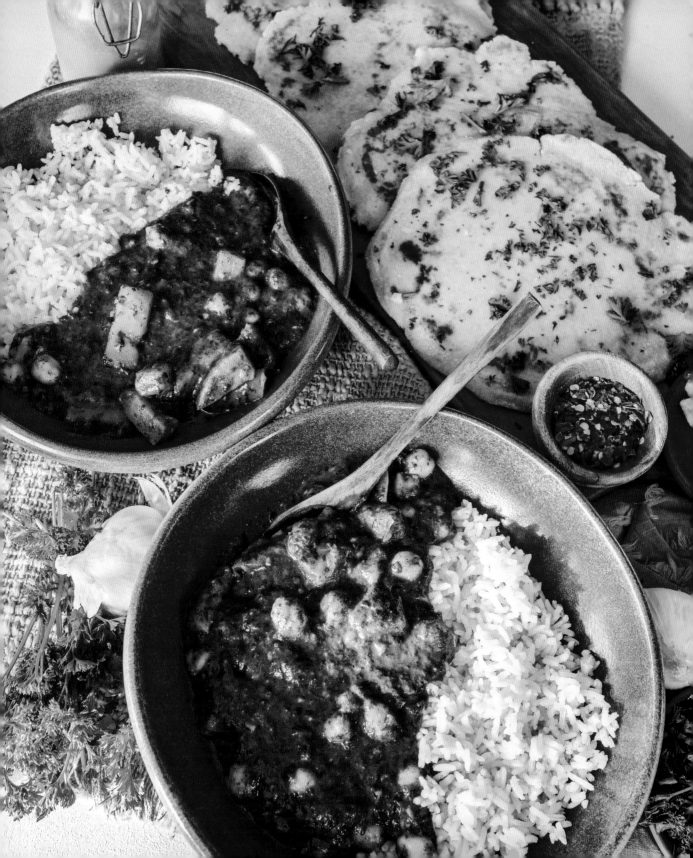

CHANA SAAG AND GLUTEN-FREE GARLIC NAAN

I have yet to find a chana saag—a creamy garbanzo bean and spinach curry—I like more than the one I make at home. This whips together faster than delivery and will easily become one of your staples! To complete the vibe, I pair the chana saag with my go-to gluten-free garlic naan bread and rice or quinoa. The naan rises while you make the saag and, quite easily, you've got fresh bread that doesn't make you bloat.

THE GOODS

GLUTEN-FREE GARLIC NAAN
1 tbsp (9 g) active dry yeast

1 tbsp (10 g) coconut sugar

½ cup (120 ml) water, warmed to about 105°F (41°C)

½ cup (120 g) unsweetened coconut yogurt

1 cup (240 ml) light or full-fat coconut milk, at room temperature

1 tsp salt

1 tsp granulated garlic

2¾ cups (330 g) cassava flour, plus more for dusting

Olive oil, as needed

CHANA SAAG
1 tsp coconut oil, melted

1 medium yellow onion, diced

1 tsp salt, divided

3 cloves garlic, minced

1 tbsp (10 g) minced fresh ginger

1 small serrano pepper, deseeded and minced

1 tsp garam masala

½ tsp ground cumin

½ tsp ground turmeric

½ tsp black pepper

2½ cups (600 ml) full-fat coconut milk

4 packed cups (400 g) baby spinach

1 (15-oz [425-g]) can garbanzo beans, drained and rinsed

2 cups (300 g) medium-diced yellow potatoes

1 cup (200 g) rice or quinoa, cooked

THE METHOD

To start the naan, combine the yeast, sugar and water in a large bowl. Let it rest for 10 minutes, until it is foamy on top. Whisk in the yogurt, milk, salt and granulated garlic. Slowly add the flour ½ cup (60 g) at a time while whisking with a fork. Once the dough becomes a ball, cover the bowl with a damp towel and let it rise for 30 to 60 minutes, until it has puffed up and is beginning to crack on top.

Meanwhile, make the chana saag. Heat the coconut oil in a large sauté pan over medium-high heat. Once hot, add the onion and ½ teaspoon of the salt. Cook for 2 to 3 minutes, until the onion begins to soften. Add the garlic, ginger and serrano pepper. Stir and cook it for 1 minute, then add the garam masala, cumin, turmeric, pepper and remaining ½ teaspoon of salt. Toast the spices and stir for 1 minute. Add the milk to deglaze the pan. Stir the mixture until it's smooth, reduce the heat to medium-low and simmer for 3 to 5 minutes. Stir in the spinach to wilt.

After about 1 minute, remove the pan from the heat and transfer the contents to a high-powered blender. Pulse the saag into a smooth and beautiful green sauce. Pour the saag back into the same sauté pan and turn the heat to medium-high. Once the saag starts to simmer, add the beans and potatoes. Cover the pan and reduce the heat to low. Simmer the saag for 10 minutes, until the potatoes are fork-tender.

While the saag is simmering, finish your naan. Pull your dough onto a floured surface, then divide it into 5 or 6 lemon-sized balls. Using a rolling pin, roll out each ball into a ½-inch (1.3-cm)-thick circle. Grab a large skillet and set it over medium-high heat. Coat the skillet with about 1 tablespoon (15 ml) of the olive oil. Sear each naan for about 30 seconds on each side, until the bread is starting to brown. You'll need to add more olive oil before flipping the naan and before adding another piece of naan, as the fat from the olive oil is crucial.

Keep the naan warm in a tortilla warmer or a basket with a clean kitchen towel. Serve the chana saag with the rice and naan.

Makes 4 servings

WATERMELON POKE BOWLS

This dish will deeply satisfy and refresh you at the same time. I always get a craving for poke when summer comes around, and the plant world really delivers here. The umami flavors of the marinade match perfectly with the sweetness of the watermelon. And the spicy sauce? Well, trust me when I say you'll want to put this sauce on everything! As important as flavor is, finding ways to enjoy sustainable seafood alternatives is even more important in our world today. Finding better alternatives to seafood consumption can not only help preserve our oceans, but it can reduce your exposure to heavy metals like mercury. Flavor and sustainability all in one dish: Watermelon poke for the win!

THE GOODS

MARINATED WATERMELON
¼ cup (60 ml) coconut aminos

2 tbsp (30 ml) toasted sesame oil

1 tbsp (15 ml) Sriracha

1 tbsp (15 ml) liquid aminos

1 tbsp (15 ml) plain rice vinegar

½ small or mini watermelon, peeled and cut into ½" (13-mm) cubes

SPICY SAUCE
½ cup (120 ml) Cashew Cream (page 173) or ½ cup (110 g) vegan mayo

1 tsp Sriracha (see Bai's Tips)

1 tsp fresh lime juice

1 tsp plain rice vinegar

POKE BOWLS
2 cups (380 g) cooked rice of choice

1 small cucumber, thinly sliced

2 small watermelon radishes, thinly sliced (see Bai's Tips)

1 large avocado, thinly sliced

1 medium carrot, shredded

1 scallion, thinly sliced

2 sheets nori, thinly sliced

1 tsp sesame seeds

1 medium lime, thickly sliced

THE METHOD

First, make the marinated watermelon. In a small Mason jar, combine the coconut aminos, oil, Sriracha, liquid aminos and vinegar. Mix the ingredients well with a fork, or secure the jar's lid and shake it until the ingredients are well combined. Place the watermelon in a large bowl and pour the marinade over the watermelon. Gently toss to cover all the watermelon in the marinade without breaking any of the little pieces. Refrigerate the watermelon for 30 minutes, or up to overnight, to infuse the watermelon with all that great flavor.

To make the spicy sauce, combine the Cashew Cream, Sriracha, lime juice and vinegar in a small bowl. Mix the ingredients well, taste the sauce for your desired spiciness and set the sauce aside.

It's time to build your poke bowls! Grab two serving bowls. First, put your rice in the bowls. Next, place a big scoop of your watermelon poke right in the middle. Add the cucumber, watermelon radishes, avocado, carrot, scallion and nori all around the watermelon poke. Sprinkle the sesame seeds on top of each serving, drizzle the poke with your spicy sauce and add the lime slices. Serve the poke bowls immediately.

BAI'S TIPS: *Add more Sriracha to the sauce if you're feelin' spicy!*

If you can't find watermelon radishes, use any variety of radish you can find.

Makes 2 servings

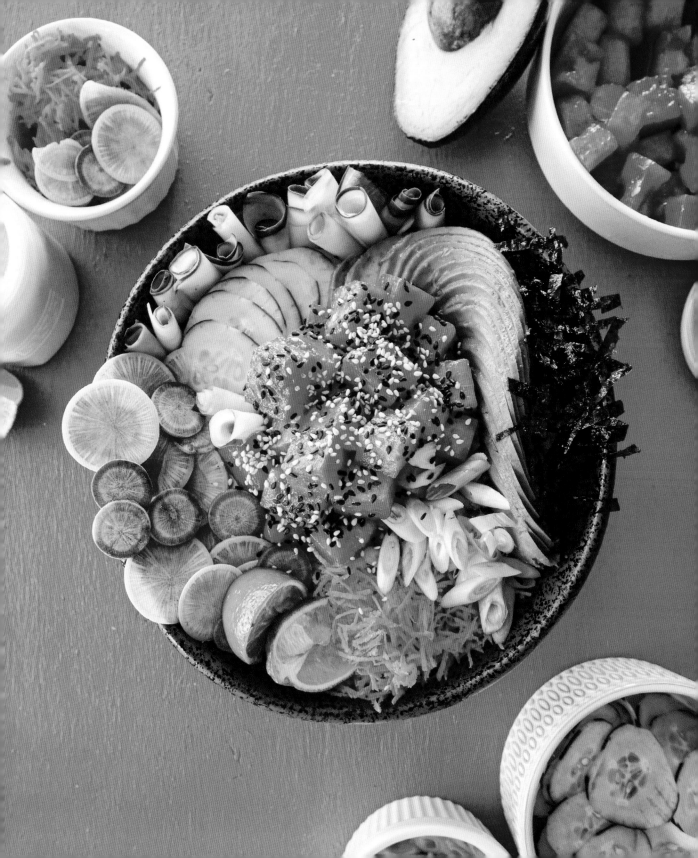

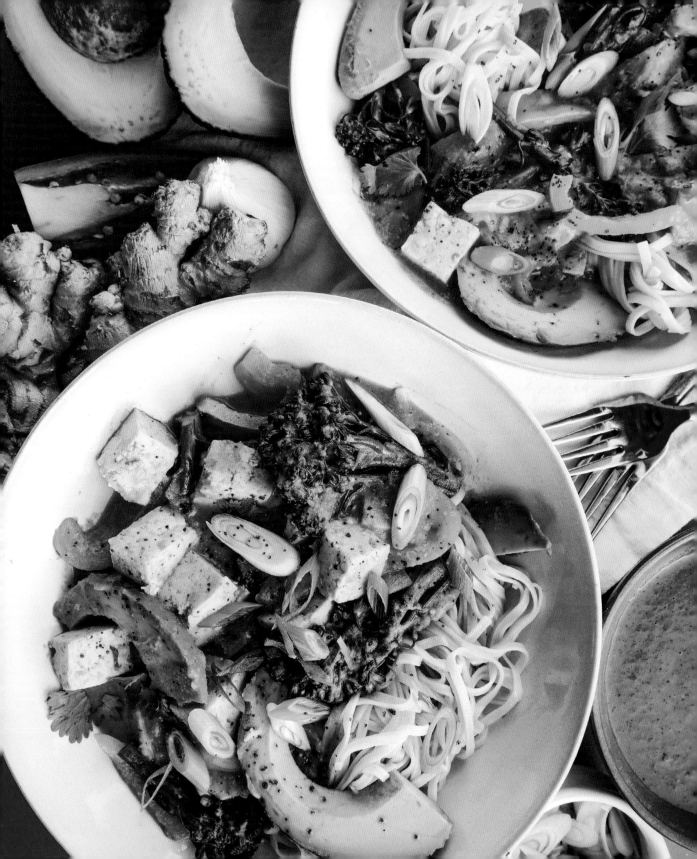

AVOCADO CURRY NOODLES

As a California girl, I always have avocados on hand in my kitchen. I eat them solo with salt, on toast, in tacos, even in chocolate mousse—but this time, they're taking on a whole new form in a Thai curry. Healthy fats like avocado and coconut milk help us absorb nutrients, are vital for brain health and are necessary when building flavor. If you're intimidated by making your own curry paste, don't be! All you do is throw a bunch of goodies into a food processor or blender and that's it. This recipe comes together quickly and is a healthy weeknight meal. In a way, this dish is just like California itself: a melting pot of diversity and full of flavor.

THE GOODS

CURRY PASTE

2 scallions, root ends removed

½ medium avocado, peeled

¼ yellow onion, chopped

¼ packed cup (30 g) fresh cilantro leaves and stems

3 cloves garlic, peeled

1 small jalapeño pepper, deseeded

1 tbsp (10 g) minced fresh ginger

¼ tsp ground cumin

¼ tsp ground coriander

¼ tsp ground turmeric

1 tbsp (15 ml) fresh lemon juice

1 tsp salt

¼ cup (60 ml) water

NOODLES

1 tsp coconut oil

¼ yellow onion, sliced

1 tsp salt, divided

1 yellow bell pepper, sliced

1 (14-oz [414-ml]) can full-fat coconut milk

1 tbsp (15 ml) liquid aminos

1 (14-oz [397-g]) block firm tofu, cut into 1" (2.5-cm) cubes

1 (8-oz [227-g]) package brown rice pad Thai noodles

1 medium bunch broccolini, destemmed

1 tbsp (15 ml) coconut aminos

2 tbsp (30 ml) fresh lime juice

1 large avocado, thickly sliced

Chopped scallions (optional)

THE METHOD

Make your curry paste first. Just toss the scallions, avocado, onion, cilantro, garlic, jalapeño, ginger, cumin, coriander, turmeric, lemon juice, salt and water into your blender or food processor and blend until the ingredients are smooth. Pour the paste into a medium bowl and set it aside.

Now make the noodles. In a large sauté pan over medium heat, combine the oil, onion and ½ teaspoon of the salt. Cook the onion for about 1 minute, until it starts to soften. Add the bell pepper and cook the vegetables for 1 minute. Add the curry paste and cook the mixture for 1 minute. Add the milk, liquid aminos and tofu. Cover the pan, turn down the heat to low and cook the curry for about 5 minutes. While this cooks, get some water boiling and cook your noodles according to the package's instructions.

Your curry should be bubbling and cooking beautifully at this point. Add your broccolini, coconut aminos, lime juice and avocado. Cover the pan and cook the curry for 5 more minutes, until the broccolini is tender and bright green. Taste the curry for spiciness and saltiness, adjusting the spiciness and adding the remaining ½ teaspoon of salt if needed.

Serve the curry in four bowls: Add the noodles to the bowls, then place the curry sauce and veggies over the top of the noodles. Garnish the curry with the scallions (if using).

BAI'S TIP: Like soup, curries tend to build flavor over time. Make the paste ahead of time, make this recipe on a meal-prep day or, at the very least, save some leftovers so you can see how the flavor develops as the curry sits for a day!

Makes 4 servings

PURPLE PESTO PIZZA

When I say, "Eat the rainbow," this recipe proves that I mean it. You're about to embark on a new journey with pizza. It's important to enter this realm with an open mind, as I designed this pizza to be different and food for fuel. Eating the rainbow is like getting nature's best multivitamin from whole-food sources. It is the absolute best way to diversify your diet and create beautiful and tasty food. Even the crust is a protein-packed and delicious way to rethink how we look at pizza dough. Preheat your oven and dive in!

THE GOODS

2¼ cups (320 g) diced purple sweet potatoes

¾ cup (90 g) cassava flour, plus more as needed

1 (15-oz [425-g]) can garbanzo beans, drained and rinsed

1 tbsp (15 g) tahini

1 tsp garlic powder

1 tsp salt

1 tbsp (15 ml) olive oil

1 cup (240 ml) Pesto (page 19), or store-bought vegan pesto

Almond Ricotta or Tofu Ricotta (page 165), or store-bought vegan ricotta

1 large heirloom tomato, cut into ¼" (6-mm)-thick slices

¼ cup (40 g) pitted Kalamata olives, sliced in half

1 tsp coarsely chopped fresh oregano

THE METHOD

First, grab a steamer basket and a large pot. Add 1 inch (2.5 cm) of water to the pot and set it over low heat. Bring the water to a boil, then add the sweet potatoes to the steamer basket and steam them for about 10 minutes, until they are fork-tender. Remove the pot from the heat, and then remove the steamer basket from the pot and set the sweet potatoes aside.

Preheat your oven to 400°F (204°C).

In a food processor, combine the sweet potatoes, flour, garbanzo beans, tahini, garlic powder, salt and oil. Process the ingredients on low speed for about 1 minute, until the dough is smooth and forms a ball.

Grab a 16-inch (40-cm) round pizza pan or a large square baking sheet and push the dough out to form a circular pizza or a square pizza, depending on your pan. You want the dough to be about ⅛ inch (3 mm) thick. If the dough sticks to your fingers, just brush some additional flour on your fingers. Note that if you have a pizza pan with holes on the bottom, you will need to put parchment paper or a silicone baking mat over the pan, press out the dough, pull the pan out from the bottom of the parchment, place the pan on top of the dough and flip the whole thing over. We want the dough directly on the pizza pan so that it can get nice and crispy on the bottom.

Bake the crust for 10 minutes. Now it's time to build our pizza! First, use a ladle to pour the Pesto all over the middle of the crust, making a thin layer. Top the Pesto with dollops of the Almond Ricotta, tomato, olives and oregano. Pop the pizza in the oven and bake it for 20 minutes, until the crust easily lifts away from the pan and the ricotta is beginning to turn golden brown.

Slide a spatula underneath the crust to release the pizza from the pizza pan, and then transfer the pizza to a cutting board. Cut the pizza into slices with a sharp knife and serve.

Makes 1 (16" [40-cm]) round pizza

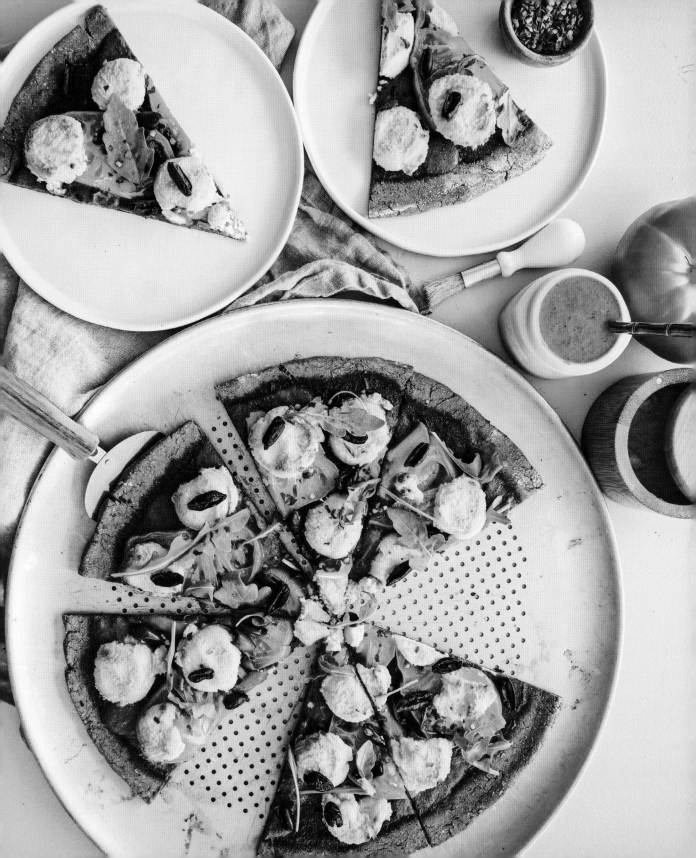

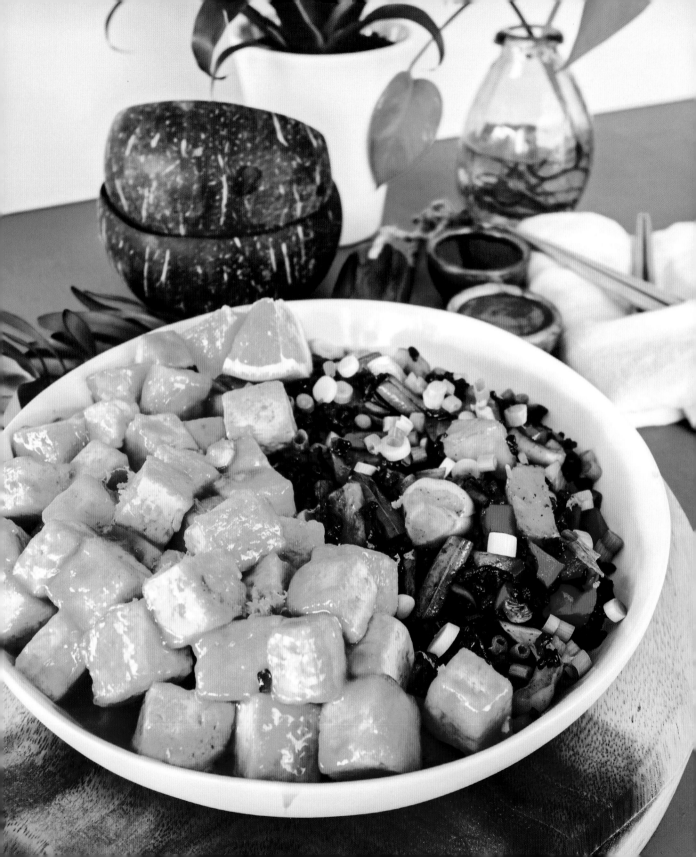

ORANGE-SESAME TOFU WITH HAWAIIAN FRIED RICE

Takeout magic delivered straight from your fridge! When I was growing up, fried rice and orange chicken were some of my favorite weekday treats, and I will admit to still regularly ordering eggless Hawaiian fried rice from my local Thai spot.

This is two delicious recipes in one, which means that it's versatile for whatever you're feelin' in the moment! The tofu and the black rice go together perfectly. Black rice is such a great alternative to brown or white rice—not just for the high protein content and antioxidant properties, but because it's textured and brings an entirely new flavor to this dish. The tofu is so flavorful and will remind you of those days you used to eat orange chicken out of a Chinese takeout box. Major yum.

THE GOODS

TOFU AND RICE

1 cup (160 g) black rice

1¾ cups (420 ml) Immune-Boosting Veggie Broth (page 170) or water

½ tsp salt

1 (14-oz [397-g]) block firm tofu, drained and pressed for at least 15 minutes (see Bai's Tips on page 133)

2 tbsp (18 g) tapioca flour

1 tbsp (15 ml) toasted sesame oil

ORANGE SAUCE

¾ cup (180 ml) fresh orange juice

2 tbsp (30 ml) toasted sesame oil

2 tbsp (30 ml) liquid aminos

1 tbsp (15 ml) coconut aminos

1 tbsp (15 ml) plain rice vinegar

1 tsp Sriracha

1 tbsp (15 ml) agave nectar

SLURRY

¼ cup (60 ml) water

1 tbsp (9 g) tapioca flour

THE METHOD

To make the tofu and rice, combine the rice, broth and salt in a small saucepan over medium-high heat. Bring the rice to a boil. Cover the saucepan and reduce the heat to medium-low. Simmer the rice for 25 to 30 minutes. When the rice is cooked, set it aside, still covered.

Cut the tofu into 1-inch (2.5-cm) cubes and toss into a medium bowl. Sprinkle the tapioca flour over the tofu and toss the tofu to make sure it gets coated—be careful not to break the tofu pieces apart.

To make the orange sauce, combine the orange juice, sesame oil, liquid aminos, coconut aminos, rice vinegar, Sriracha and agave in a medium Mason jar. Stir the ingredients with a fork until the sauce is smooth. Set the sauce aside.

Heat a large, nontoxic nonstick sauté pan over medium-high heat and add the sesame oil. Once the oil is hot, add the tofu. Sear the tofu for 2 minutes on each side, until it's crispy and golden brown—this should take about 9 to 12 minutes total. Pour the orange sauce over the tofu and stir to coat the tofu in the sauce. Cook the tofu and sauce for 2 to 3 minutes, and meanwhile make the slurry: In a small bowl, combine the water and tapioca flour. Add the slurry to the tofu and cook the tofu for 2 minutes, stirring it constantly—you'll see the sauce thicken quite quickly. Remove the pan from the heat, cover it and set it aside.

(continued)

FRIED RICE

1 tbsp (15 ml) melted coconut oil

2 cups (220 g) 1" (2.5 cm)-long pieces green beans

1 cup (140 g) finely chopped fresh pineapple

1 medium bunch bok choy, thickly sliced

1 medium red bell pepper, coarsely chopped

2 tbsp (30 ml) liquid aminos

1 tbsp (15 ml) coconut aminos

1 tsp granulated garlic

2 scallions, coarsely chopped, plus more as needed

Orange zest, as needed (optional)

Orange slices, as needed (optional)

As the tofu is doing its thing, heat the coconut oil in a separate large sauté pan over medium-high heat. Once the coconut oil is hot, toss in the green beans, pineapple, bok choy and bell pepper. Cook the vegetables for 1 minute, stirring them constantly. Add the liquid aminos, coconut aminos and granulated garlic. Cook the mixture for 2 to 3 minutes, stirring it constantly. Finally, add all of the cooked black rice, mix everything together and cook the fried rice for 3 minutes. In the last 30 seconds of cooking, add the scallions and toss everything together.

To serve, you can use either a large serving plate or three or four serving bowls. Plate the fried rice, and then top it with the tofu and drizzle everything with the leftover sauce. Garnish the dish with more scallions, the orange zest (if using) and oranges slices (if using) if you're feeling extra frisky! Serve this dish immediately or make it as your meal prep, as it makes great leftovers!

BAI'S TIP: You can use any rice—or even quinoa—for this recipe. Just make sure to cook it according to the package's instructions. I love the color and texture of black rice, but you do you! If you want to heat up leftovers, just add a bit of sesame oil or veggie broth to a pan, add your leftovers and toss them until they are heated through. If your rice got really dried out in the fridge, add another splash of veggie broth and a dash of coconut aminos.

Makes 3 to 4 servings

CHICAGO-STYLE CLASSIC DEEP-DISH PIZZA

Hellooo, gorgeous pizza! Chicago deep-dish speaks for itself with all that messy cheesiness. My father, a New Yorker, would be upset at this dedication to one of the best ways to eat pizza. But I'm pretty sure my husband, a Chicagoan, married me for this recipe, so you know it was worth the switch in loyalty. This deep-dish pizza comes with no food coma, no BS and no cruelty. Made entirely with plants, this is something we vegans only dreamed about for a long time—but now that it's here in its physical form, there's no going back. And I couldn't just give you a basic pizza! This is a pizza with a spelt crust, freshly made mozzarella, caramelized onions, mushrooms, peppers, a whole lotta basil and fire-roasted tomatoes. It's the Michael Jordan of vegan pizza, the cream of the crop—you know, the Sears Tower. Your world is about to be changed, and I'm just glad to be here for it.

THE GOODS

CRUST
1 tbsp (9 g) active dry yeast

1 tbsp (10 g) coconut sugar

1 cup (240 ml) water, warmed to about 105°F (41°C)

3 tbsp (45 ml) olive oil

1 tsp salt

2¼ cups (360 g) spelt flour, plus more as needed

MOZZARELLA CHEESE
1 cup (150 g) raw cashews, soaked in cool water for 6 hours or in hot water for 15 minutes and drained

1¼ cups (300 ml) water

½ tsp garlic powder

½ tsp salt

1 tsp nutritional yeast

1 tsp miso paste

3 tbsp (27 g) tapioca flour

THE METHOD

First, make the crust. In a large bowl, combine the yeast, sugar and water, but do not stir the ingredients. Let the mixture sit for about 5 minutes. The hot water will activate the yeast while the yeast feeds on the sugar. You'll know it's bloomed and ready when there is a layer of foam on the top. Once you see the foamy layer, add the oil and mix everything together. Then add the salt and the spelt flour 1 cup (160 g) at a time while continuing to mix. I mix the dough with a fork at first, but you can use a stand mixer with the dough attachment. Once the dough has formed, I like to switch to kneading with my hands. The dough should not stick to your hands, and it should bounce back when touched. When it reaches this stage, stop kneading it. Cover it with a damp kitchen towel and let it rise for 30 to 45 minutes.

While your dough is doing its thing, get your mozzarella cheese ready. In a blender, combine the cashews, water, garlic powder, salt, nutritional yeast, miso and tapioca flour. Blend the ingredients on high speed for 30 to 45 seconds, until the mixture is smooth and creamy. Pour the mozzarella into a cold medium saucepan. Heat the mozzarella over medium-low heat while stirring it constantly with a rubber spatula for 8 minutes. Make sure the mozzarella doesn't burn or stick to the bottom of the saucepan. If it starts to burn or stick, reduce the heat or remove the saucepan from the heat completely for a few seconds to let it cool down a little. You'll see the mozzarella start to thicken like magic a few moments before it's done. Once it's thick and gooey, remove it from the heat and set it aside.

(continued)

VEGGIES

1 tbsp (15 ml) olive oil

1 small onion, thinly sliced

½ tsp salt

½ tsp black pepper

½ tsp coconut sugar

3 cups (240 g) thinly sliced cremini mushrooms

1 cup (100 g) thinly sliced sweet peppers

1 cup (30 g) coarsely chopped fresh basil, divided

2 cups (60 g) baby spinach

1 (15-oz [425-g]) can diced fire-roasted tomatoes, undrained, or 2 large tomatoes, coarsely chopped

Prep your veggies by grabbing a 10-inch (25-cm) sauté pan—for best results, use a cast-iron pan—and heat the oil over medium-high heat. Add the onion and salt and cook the onion for 3 to 4 minutes, stirring it frequently. Add the black pepper and sugar—the sugar will help the onion caramelize. Cook the onion for 2 minutes, stirring it frequently. Add the mushrooms and sweet peppers. Cook the veggies for 5 minutes, stirring them frequently. All the veggies should be softened, and the mushrooms should be starting to turn brown. Add the basil—saving about 1 tablespoon (2 g) for the top of the pizza—and the spinach. Cook the mixture for 2 minutes, stirring it constantly, until the spinach has softened and wilted. Remove the pan from the heat and set it aside.

Preheat the oven to 400°F (204°C) and grab a 10-inch (25-cm) cast-iron sauté pan—you can use the same pan you cooked the veggies in; just be sure to clean it and oil it before using it again.

Lightly punch down the dough. Clean your work surface and dust it with flour. Remove the dough from the bowl. Knead it five or six times, and then roll it out to a circle with a rolling pin. Once it's a bit bigger than the size of your pan, carefully transfer the dough to the pan. If you rip it, that's okay—because it's a deep-dish crust, it's forgiving. Just patch it up and keep moving forward. Lay the dough evenly in the pan and press it up the pan's sides, so the dough is an even thickness throughout.

Add the mozzarella first by spreading it all on the bottom and halfway up the sides of the crust. Next, add the veggies and the fire-roasted tomatoes with their juices. I like to then slightly roll the crust in on itself about ½ inch (1.3 cm) to seal the deal. Bake the pizza for 25 to 30 minutes, or until the crust is light brown on the top and is hard to the touch.

Remove the pizza from the oven, sprinkle the reserved basil on the top of the pizza and let it cool for 10 minutes before cutting it, so that everything inside can set. You can remove the entire thing from the pan and then cut it, or you can cut it inside the pan—it's up to you!

Makes 1 (10-inch [25-cm]) pizza

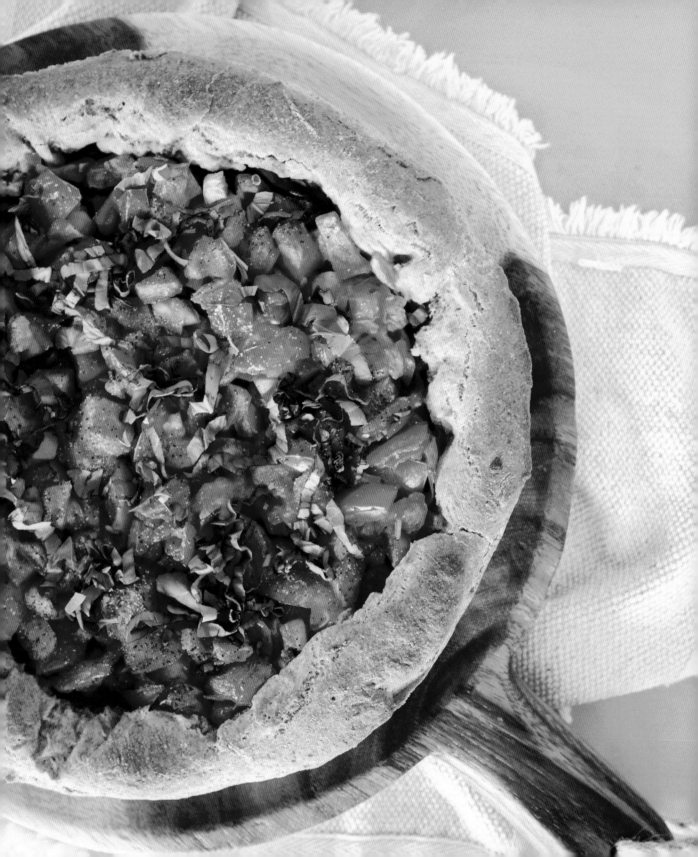

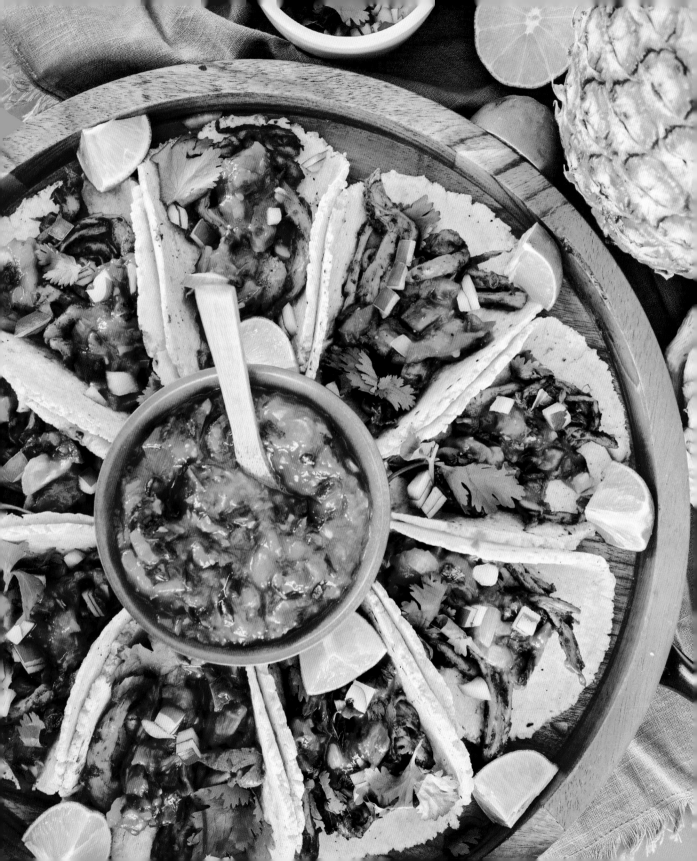

INSPIRED BY *Mexico*

I spent a good chunk of my twenties traveling to and around Mexico. The culture is not my own, but it is a culture I respect, cherish and have learned so much from—I felt an entire chapter needed to be dedicated to honoring the lessons, cooking techniques, amazing people and culture I experienced in Mexico. It may seem like Mexican food would be hard to veganize, but in reality, it is the perfect place to start.

Mexican produce and recipes are filled with colors, flavors and intention. When you look closely, you can see the attention to detail on so many things. The ingredients, spices and flavor combinations are the ideal starting point for vegan dishes, because a lot of Mexican cuisine is actually made out of plants! Examples of this are the salsas, guacamoles, spices, verde sauces and citrus used in Mexican food to create depth of flavor.

What strikes me the most about this culture in comparison to what we experience in the US is the fact that family is the most important thing, and that emphasis on family spills over into how Mexican people experience food. Grandmothers are still teaching their grand-children and great grandchildren how to make things like tamales, fresh cheese, mole sauce, tortillas and salsa. It's a culture deeply rooted in tradition that, in my experience, focuses on the comfort and immense flavor food can bring. To keep recipes alive, we depend on the older generation to teach us, which is something I feel we're losing here in the States.

I have a lot to learn about this culture and still have so many corners of Mexico to travel to. The areas I have traveled to have expanded my mind as a person and as a chef in ways I never thought possible. The Mayan Riviera taught me how to relax and about the importance of fresh ceviche and a margarita under a palm tree. Baja California taught me to honor simplicity; showed me the key to an amazing salsa; taught me how to make a carajillo; and helped me realize that Pacifico beer is truly better than Tecate® beer. Oaxaca taught me that mezcal is the best spirit in the world. And finally, Guadalajara taught me that family and good food are rooted in healing and happiness.

Whatever your experience of Mexican food, I urge you to cook through this chapter with a fresh mind and eagerness to try Mexican cuisine in a whole new way. Every recipe has been made with intention not only to help you experience this culture in a plant-based way but also to help you become the badass cook that I know you can be. You'll make "meat" out of plants like king oyster mushrooms (page 66) and hibiscus (page 73). You'll be transported to a taqueria with Tacos Al Pastor (page 61). You'll gain a new breakfast obsession with Chilaquiles (page 77), and you'll make salsas that work for any occasion (page 61, page 70 and page 77). Welcome to the world of vegan Mexican food—you'll never be the same.

Salud!

CAULIFLOWER-AVOCADO CEVICHE

Ceviche reminds me of sitting on a beach chair in Mexico, watching the waves in the middle of the afternoon, drinking a margarita and just full-on living the dream. Ceviche is as fresh as it gets! It's cooked by the acidity in the lemon and lime juices, making this a no-heat recipe that just takes a bit of chopping and marinating. You can still get the tropical feel of ceviche without the fish! The cauliflower softens in the acidity and is the perfect replacement for seafood. The tomatillos, fresh orange juice, strawberries, garlic and bell pepper make for an incredible flavor combination. Make sure to check out my tip at the end of the recipe to make chips too—they're not only tasty, but they also use less salt and oil, making them a much healthier alternative to typical corn chips. So go on, make some ceviche, pair it with a margarita, kick your feet up, soak up the sun and live the dream!

THE GOODS

3 cups (300 g) cauliflower florets, finely chopped

1 (15-oz [425-g]) can pinto beans, drained and rinsed

1 medium red onion, finely chopped

12 strawberries, tops removed and coarsely chopped

1 large red bell pepper, coarsely chopped

1 large tomatillo, finely chopped

1 medium jalapeño pepper, deseeded and minced

1 large avocado, diced

2 radishes, thinly sliced

3 cloves garlic, minced

1 packed cup (120 g) fresh cilantro, finely chopped

1 to 2 tsp salt, divided

½ cup (120 ml) fresh orange juice

½ cup (120 ml) fresh lime juice

¼ cup (60 ml) fresh lemon juice

THE METHOD

In a large serving bowl, combine the cauliflower, beans, onion, strawberries, bell pepper, tomatillo, jalapeño, avocado, radishes, garlic, cilantro, 1 teaspoon of the salt, orange juice, lime juice and lemon juice. Mix the ingredients together for 2 minutes to make sure they are well combined. Cover the bowl, transfer it to the refrigerator and allow the ceviche to marinate for 1 hour, or preferably overnight.

Once your ceviche has marinated, taste it for salt and add the remaining 1 teaspoon of salt if you feel like it needs extra seasoning.

BAI'S TIPS: If you'd like to make homemade chips, preheat your oven to 375°F (191°C). Cut 6 cassava or corn tortillas into triangles—you can do this easily by stacking them up and then cutting them like a pizza. In a large bowl, toss your tortilla triangles with 1 tablespoon (15 ml) of olive oil and a healthy pinch of salt. Place the triangles on a large baking sheet and bake them for 10 minutes. Pull them out of the oven, toss them and return them to the oven. Bake them for 3 to 4 minutes, until they are crispy. Enjoy your crispy chips with the ceviche!

Make this dish for meal prep by letting the ceviche marinate in the bowl for 30 minutes and then dividing it between widemouthed Mason jars. Let the ceviche marinate overnight, and then take it to work with you throughout the week. It will stay good for 5 to 6 days.

Makes 4 servings

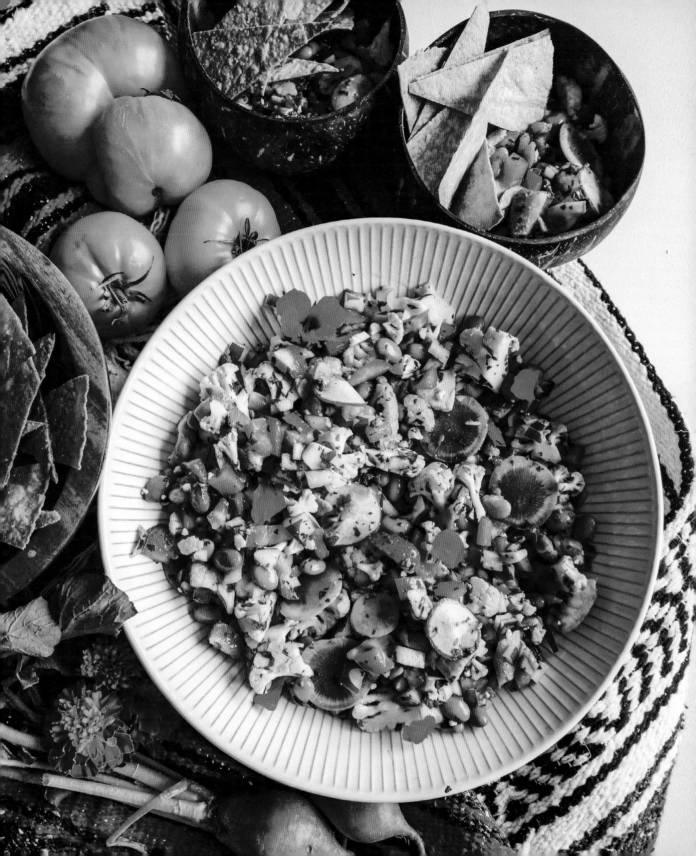

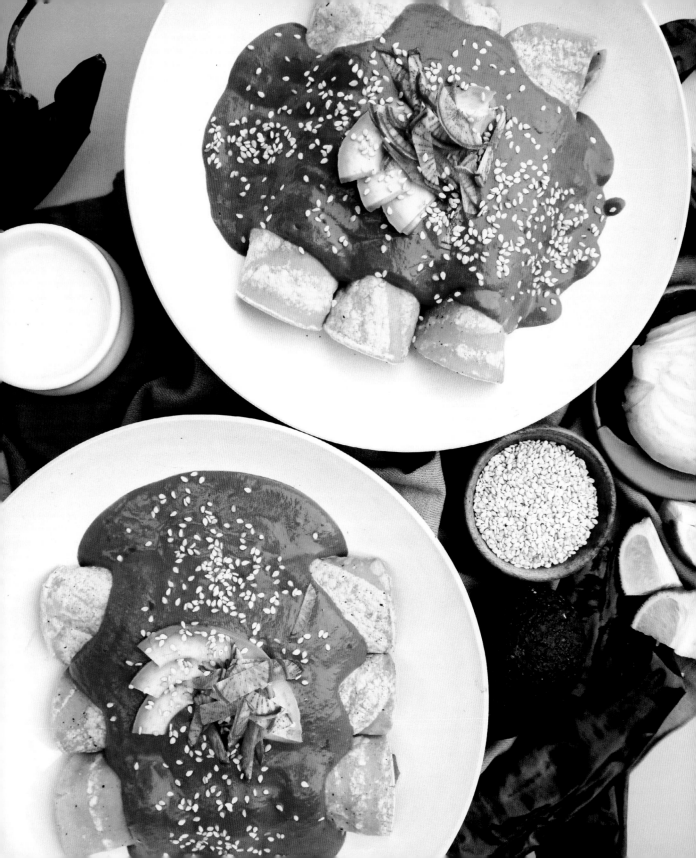

MOLE FAMILY-STYLE ENCHILADAS

Whenever I see mole on the menu of an authentic Mexican restaurant, you better believe I'm ordering it! Mole is one of the most sacred and well-kept secrets of many Mexican families and chefs. So much so that I thought a lot about whether I should include it in this collection of recipes. There is even a mole by chef Enrique Olvera that is cooked for more than 1,400 days that I am hoping to try one day. This quick sauce is no 1,400-day mole, but it can help you experience some of the joy of creating a complex mole sauce wherever in the world you are cooking. It's so delicious on these enchiladas or by itself with fresh tortillas (page 62). I truly believe that sauces are the key to cuisine, and vegan cuisine is no exception to this rule. Sauces should not be overlooked, especially one like mole or enchilada sauce in general. If mole is way outside of your comfort zone, take that as a sign that you need to make this recipe. Ditch the canned sauce, grab some guajillo chilies and dive into these enchiladas. You'll be so glad you did.

THE GOODS

MOLE

1 tsp olive oil

2 to 3 large guajillo chilies, finely chopped

1 medium onion, finely chopped

Salt, as needed

4 cloves garlic, minced

4 medium tomatillos, quartered

½ tsp ground cumin

½ tsp ground coriander

½ tsp ground cinnamon

½ tsp paprika

¼ tsp ground cloves

2½ to 3 cups (600 to 720 ml) Immune-Boosting Veggie Broth (page 170), divided

¼ cup (60 g) tahini

2 tbsp (30 g) smooth almond butter

½ cup (120 g) diced fresh tomatoes or 2 heaping tbsp (50 g) tomato paste

3 tbsp (45 ml) pure maple syrup

¼ cup (30 g) cacao powder

THE METHOD

First, make the mole. In a deep sauté pan over medium-high heat, combine the oil and guajillo chilies. Cook them for 2 minutes, then toss in the onion and a pinch of salt. Sauté the mixture for 2 minutes, until the onion softens.

Next, add the garlic and cook the mixture for 1 minute. Throw in the tomatillos, cumin, coriander, cinnamon, paprika and cloves and sauté the mixture for 1 minute. Once the crust on the bottom of the pan is crispy and almost burned, pour in ½ cup (120 ml) of the broth and the tahini. Mix the ingredients together and reduce the heat to medium. Cook the mixture for 1 minute. Add 1 cup (240 ml) of the broth, cover the pan and cook the mixture for 3 to 4 minutes. Uncover the pan and mix in the almond butter, tomatoes, maple syrup, cacao, 1 cup (240 ml) of the broth and a pinch of salt. Mix the ingredients together evenly. Cook the mole down for 3 minutes, add a last pinch of salt and remove the pan from the heat. Once the mole has cooled a bit, transfer it to a blender and puree it. Depending on your preference, you can add the remaining ½ cup (120 ml) of broth now and blend it with the mole if you want the mole to be thinner.

(continued)

ENCHILADAS

1 tsp olive oil

1 medium onion, finely chopped

¼ tsp salt

1 medium orange bell pepper, diced

2 cloves garlic, diced

2 tbsp (10 g) nutritional yeast

2 (15-oz [425-g]) cans black beans, drained and rinsed

2 medium yellow potatoes, diced

½ cup (120 ml) Immune-Boosting Veggie Broth (page 170)

14 corn tortillas

TOPPINGS

Thinly sliced avocadoes

Thinly sliced radishes

Sesame seeds

Now it's time to make the enchiladas. In another large sauté pan over medium-high heat, combine the oil, onion and salt. Cook the onion for 1 minute, then add the bell pepper and garlic. Cook the mixture for 1 minute. Add the nutritional yeast, beans, potatoes and broth. Cover the pan and reduce the heat to medium-low. Cook the mixture for 10 minutes. Uncover the pan and cook the mixture for 5 minutes to allow the liquid to evaporate. Taste the mixture to check its seasoning and the doneness of the potatoes—they should be fork-tender.

Preheat the oven to 350°F (177°C).

While the oven preheats, prepare your tortillas if they aren't fresh. Cook them on your stovetop—either in a medium skillet or directly over a flame—for 30 seconds on each side. Put the hot tortillas in a basket, then cover them up, so that their heat creates steam to soften them.

Pour about ½ cup (120 ml) of the mole sauce on the bottom of a 9 x 13–inch (23 x 33–cm) baking dish. Place about ¼ cup (60 g) of the bean and potato mixture into a tortilla, and then roll the tortilla around the filling to make an enchilada. Place the enchilada in a line in the baking dish. Continue this process until all the filling is rolled into the tortillas. Top the enchiladas with the remaining mole sauce, cover the baking dish with an ovenproof lid and bake the enchiladas for 20 to 25 minutes, until the sauce is bubbling and the edges have browned.

To serve the enchiladas, grab a few plates and place three enchiladas on each plate. Top the enchiladas with the avocadoes, radishes and sesame seeds.

BAI'S TIPS: The number of guajillo chilies you use will depend on how spicy you like your food: Use 2 chilies for a mild mole and 3 to 4 chilies for a spicy one!

Once you get this recipe down, start playing with the mole by adding more or less of different ingredients. Mole is as unique as each of us, and this is a great opportunity to experiment and create your own version!

Makes 14 enchiladas

TACOS AL PASTOR

Here's a little taste of Mexican street food right in your own kitchen. The interesting history with al pastor is that it actually originated from Lebanese immigrants who introduced Mexico to shawarma. So basically, this is my plant-based version of the Mexican version of Lebanese shawarma. Although this recipe is the furthest thing from cooking meat on a stick, small oyster mushrooms provide the texture and flexibility to give you almost the exact same texture and flavor of slowly roasted pork. It takes only a fraction of the time and a fraction of the environmental resources. On top of all that goodness, this is three recipes in one—I just couldn't help myself! Nothing beats a lunch off a taco stand with fresh homemade tortillas, roasted mango salsa and crispy al pastor–style tacos, and now you can have it from any corner of the world.

THE GOODS

TACO MEAT

1 cup (140 g) chopped pineapple

1 tsp paprika

½ tsp ground cumin

½ tsp salt

½ tsp black pepper

½ tsp chipotle powder or 1 tbsp (15 g) minced canned chipotle peppers in adobo sauce

1 tbsp (3 g) finely chopped fresh oregano or dried oregano

¼ tsp ground cloves

½ tsp granulated garlic

¼ cup (60 ml) white wine vinegar

¼ cup (60 ml) fresh orange juice

1 tbsp (15 ml) olive oil

12 oz (340 g) oyster mushrooms

SALSA

1 medium poblano pepper, deseeded and diced

1 medium yellow onion, diced

1 medium mango, peeled and diced

3 large tomatoes or 2 cups (300 g) cherry tomatoes, quartered

3 cloves garlic, peeled

1 medium jalapeño pepper, deseeded

1 tsp olive oil

½ packed cup (60 g) fresh cilantro leaves

2 tbsp (30 ml) fresh lime juice

1 tsp salt

THE METHOD

First, make the taco meat. In a high-powered blender, combine the pineapple, paprika, cumin, salt, black pepper, chipotle powder, oregano, cloves, granulated garlic, vinegar, orange juice and oil. Blend the ingredients for 20 seconds, until they are smooth. Set the sauce aside.

Grab your mushrooms and shred them with your fingers into smaller pieces. Put them in a large bowl and pour the sauce over the mushrooms. Mix everything together until the mushrooms are fully coated. Cover the bowl, transfer it to the refrigerator and marinate the mushrooms for at least 30 minutes—the longer, the better.

As the mushrooms marinate, make the salsa. Preheat your oven to a high broil. Place the poblano, yellow onion, mango, tomatoes, garlic and jalapeño on a large baking sheet. Drizzle the oil over the mixture and shake the baking sheet until everything is lightly coated with oil. Roast the mixture for 12 to 15 minutes, until the onions are crispy and the tomatoes are soft. Transfer the mixture to a blender, and then add the cilantro, lime juice and salt. Pulse the ingredients 15 to 20 times to create the salsa. If you like it chunky, then pulse the blender only a few times; or if you like a smoother consistency, pulse the blender more. Set the salsa aside.

(continued)

TORTILLAS
1 cup (120 g) cassava flour
1 cup (100 g) masa flour
1 tsp salt
1 tbsp (15 ml) olive oil
1¼ cups (300 ml) water

GARNISHES
Finely chopped red onion
Finely chopped fresh cilantro
Lime wedges

As the goods for the salsa cook, make the tortillas. Grab a large bowl and mix together the cassava flour, masa flour and salt with a fork. Add the oil and then slowly add the water ½ cup (120 ml) at a time. Mix the dough with your fork until it comes together, then use your hands and form it into a ball until the texture becomes spongy and soft. You don't want the dough to be wet, but you also don't want it to fall apart if you create a ball with it. Let the dough rest for 10 minutes.

Slice the dough into eight to ten smaller pieces, then form each piece into a ball. Create eight balls if you are looking for a bigger taco or ten if you want a smaller street-style taco. Line a tortilla press with parchment paper. If you don't have a tortilla press, you can use a rolling pin or the bottom of a plate to press the dough between two pieces of parchment paper. Press the tortillas carefully with the tortilla press.

Heat a dry large skillet over medium-high heat. Place the tortillas in the skillet and dry-cook them for 30 to 60 seconds on each side. Each side is done when it can slide easily around the skillet, kind of like an air hockey puck. Once each tortilla is done, place it immediately in a tortilla warmer or a large bowl lined with a clean kitchen towel. Cover the tortillas to keep them warm—this is important, as it allows the tortillas to steam after being cooked; otherwise they will fall apart. Let them steam inside the warmer for at least 5 minutes. Set the tortillas aside.

Now that the mushrooms have marinated, heat a medium cast-iron or steel skillet over medium-high heat. Once the skillet is hot, shake the excess marinade from the mushrooms and cook the mushrooms for 7 to 10 minutes, stirring them occasionally with tongs, until the marinade has evaporated and the mushrooms are beginning to get brown and crispy.

Now it is time to assemble your tacos. Grab a big serving platter or individual serving plates and place the tortillas on the platter or plates. Add the mushrooms to each tortilla, then some salsa. Finish off each taco by garnishing it with the red onion, cilantro and lime wedges. Serve the tacos immediately.

BAI'S TIP: Making your own tortillas is actually quite simple and worth the bit of extra effort! You can get a tortilla press for fewer than ten dollars online or at your local Mexican supermarket, and it truly does make all the difference. If you don't have time to make your own, store-bought tortillas work great too.

Makes 8 to 10 tacos

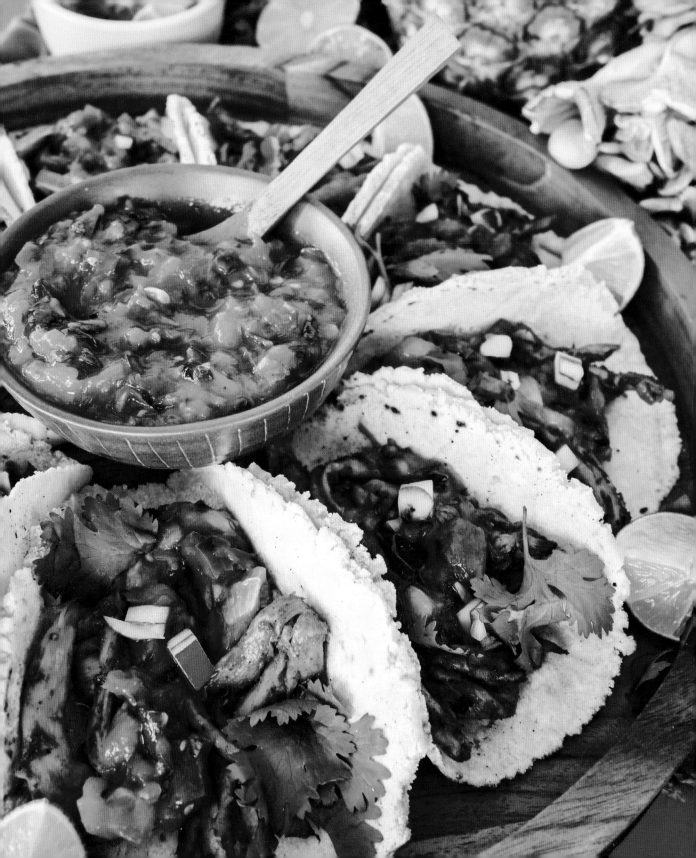

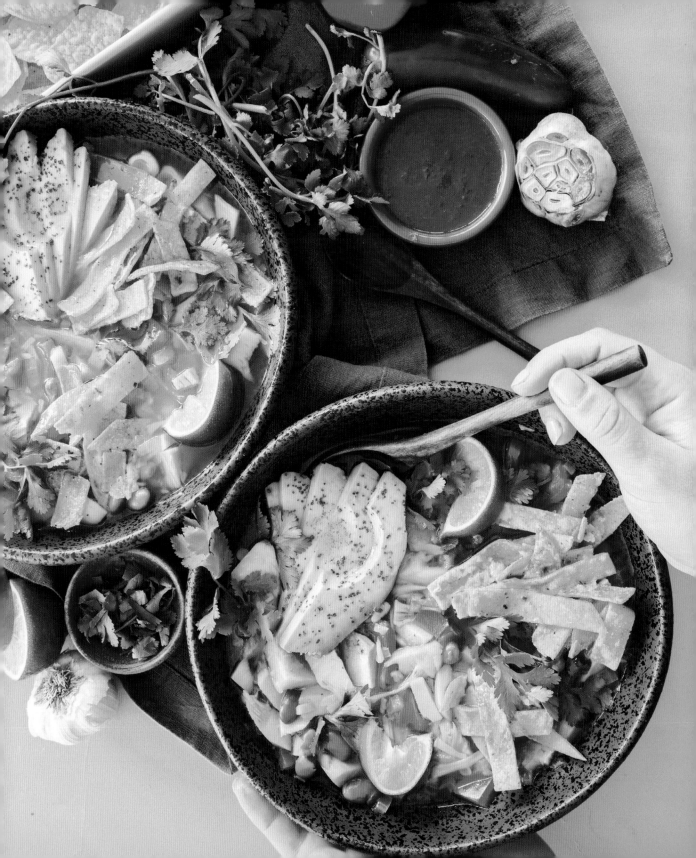

JACKFRUIT TORTILLA SOUP

A bowl of tortilla soup can make you feel—even if only for that moment—that everything is good in the world. My bestie from culinary school, Paulina Sol, who is now a restaurant owner, was the first to teach me about real Mexican comfort food. Her family took me to Guadalajara during one of my severe episodes of chronic illness and taught me the power of healing through this culture. Their restaurant Vive Sol in Mountain View, California, has one of the most incredible tortilla soups I've ever had. This recipe is dedicated to Paulina's family and highlights the fresh ingredients and spices I love most about Mexican food. It's all about simple ingredients, positive energy, a bit of spice and a whole lotta love.

THE GOODS

1 tsp plus 1 tbsp (15 ml) olive oil, divided (see Bai's Tip)

1 medium yellow onion, thinly sliced

Pinch plus ½ tsp salt, divided, plus more as needed

3 cloves garlic, minced

1 tsp ground cumin

1 tsp ground coriander

½ tsp black pepper

5 cups (1.2 L) Immune-Boosting Veggie Broth (page 170), divided

1 medium serrano pepper, deseeded and diced

1 large red bell pepper, thinly sliced

1 (15-oz [425-g]) can pinto beans, drained and rinsed

2 (20-oz [567-g]) cans jackfruit, drained, rinsed and coarsely chopped

6 small corn or wheat tortillas, sliced into thin strips

2 tbsp (30 ml) fresh lime juice

1 medium avocado, thinly sliced,

Finely chopped fresh cilantro, as needed

Cashew Cream (page 173), for topping

THE METHOD

Heat 1 teaspoon of the oil in a large pot over medium-high heat. Toss in the onion and the pinch of salt. Sauté the onion for 2 to 3 minutes, and then add the garlic, cumin, coriander, black pepper and remaining ½ teaspoon of salt. Mix the ingredients until everything is coated with the spices. Cook the mixture for 2 to 3 minutes; it will start to toast and brown on the bottom of the pot. If needed, add ¼ cup (60 ml) of the broth to deglaze the pot. Then add the serrano pepper and bell pepper and cook the mixture for 1 to 2 minutes. Add the beans and jackfruit. Stir the mixture to coat them with the spices and toast the mixture for 1 to 2 minutes. Add the remaining 4¾ cups (1.1 L) of broth. Cover the pot, reduce the heat to medium-low and cook the soup for 10 to 15 minutes.

As the soup cooks, heat the remaining 1 tablespoon (15 ml) of oil in a small sauté pan over medium-high heat. Toss in the tortilla strips and cook them for 3 to 4 minutes, until they are crispy. Set the tortilla strips aside.

Add the lime juice to the soup. Taste it for salt and add additional salt if needed. Cook the soup for 5 to 10 minutes, then remove it from the heat.

Serve the soup with the avocado, cilantro, Cashew Cream and tortilla strips.

BAI'S TIP: *If you prefer, you can air-fry the tortillas for oil-free tortilla strips!*

Makes 3 to 4 servings

CRISPY CARNITAS MUSHROOM BURRITOS

Living in San Diego means that you indulge in a burrito at least once a week. Since burritos are acceptable to eat any time of the day, it's very important to have access to a ridiculously delicious burrito wherever in the world you are. That is why this recipe is a must-have! The crispy carnitas mushrooms make this recipe unique, but they still satisfy all the cravings. If you are just starting your plant-based journey, this recipe is going to hit the spot. Enjoy the carnitas alone on a salad, on Chilaquiles (page 77), in tacos and anywhere else your heart desires!

THE GOODS

CARNITAS MUSHROOMS
3 large king oyster mushrooms
⅓ cup (80 ml) coconut aminos
¼ tsp chipotle powder
½ tsp smoked paprika
½ tsp ground cumin
½ tsp ground coriander
½ tsp granulated garlic
½ tsp salt

PICO DE GALLO
4 large heirloom tomatoes, diced into medium pieces
½ small red onion, diced
½ tsp salt
1 medium jalapeño pepper, deseeded and minced
2 tbsp (30 ml) fresh lime juice
2 cloves garlic, minced

BURRITOS
1 (15-oz [425-g]) can black beans, drained and rinsed
2 large tortillas
¼ cup (60 ml) Cashew Cream (page 173) or vegan sour cream (optional)
1 medium radish, thickly sliced
1 large avocado, thinly sliced
1 large orange or yellow bell pepper, coarsely chopped
¼ cup (12 g) finely chopped fresh cilantro (optional)

THE METHOD

First, begin preparing the carnitas mushrooms. Grab your gorgeous mushrooms and peel them into pieces lengthwise, starting from the bottom, like you would with string cheese. Once you've shredded them, place the mushrooms in a medium bowl. Drizzle the coconut aminos over the top of the mushrooms. Add the chipotle powder, smoked paprika, cumin, coriander, granulated garlic and salt. Mix the mushrooms well with a fork or your hands to make sure they are all coated with the coconut aminos and spices. Allow the mushrooms to marinate at room temperature for 20 to 40 minutes.

Make your pico de gallo while your mushrooms are marinating. In a medium bowl, mix together the tomatoes, onion, salt, jalapeño, lime juice and garlic. Taste the pico de gallo and adjust the seasonings as needed. Set it aside.

After the mushrooms have marinated, heat a medium skillet over medium-high heat. Remove the mushrooms from the marinade, saving the marinade juices for the beans, and add the mushrooms to the skillet. Cook them for 8 to 10 minutes, stirring them frequently, until they are crispy on the outside and soft on the inside. Don't let these burn! Remove the mushrooms from the skillet and set them aside.

To make the burritos, place the same skillet over medium-high heat. Add the beans and the reserved marinade. Cook the beans for 2 minutes, stirring them frequently, until all the marinade is absorbed. Set the beans aside.

Now it's time to assemble your burritos. In the middle of a tortilla, add some of the Cashew Cream (if using). Top the Cashew Cream with half of the carnitas and half of the beans. Add the radish, avocado, bell pepper, cilantro and pico de gallo. Roll the bottom of the tortilla up around the goods inside first, then fold the sides of the tortilla toward the inside to keep everything secure, and then finish by rolling the tortilla all the way up. Repeat with the other tortilla. If you are taking the burritos with you on the go, wrap each in parchment paper and enjoy them anytime, anywhere.

Makes 2 burritos

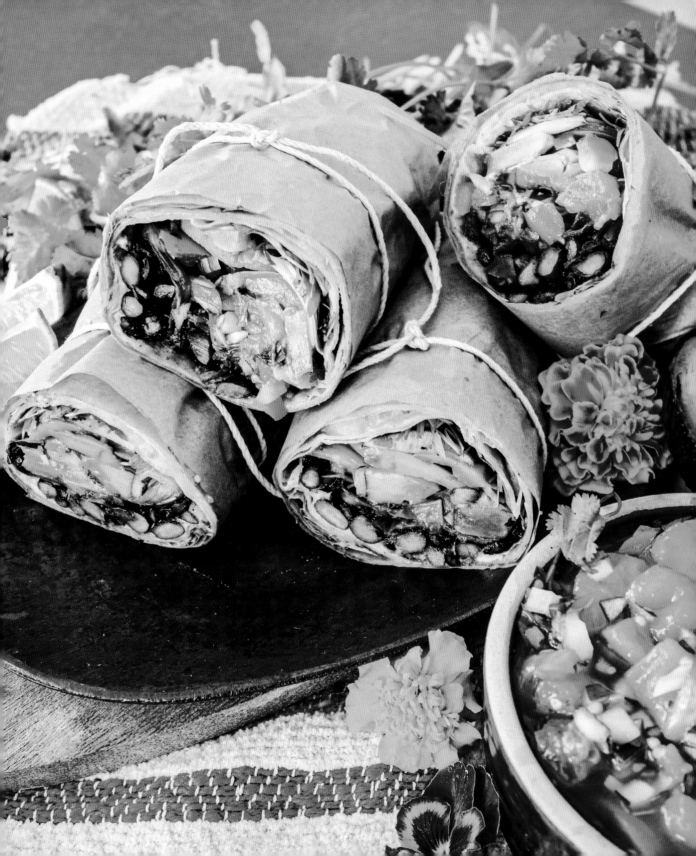

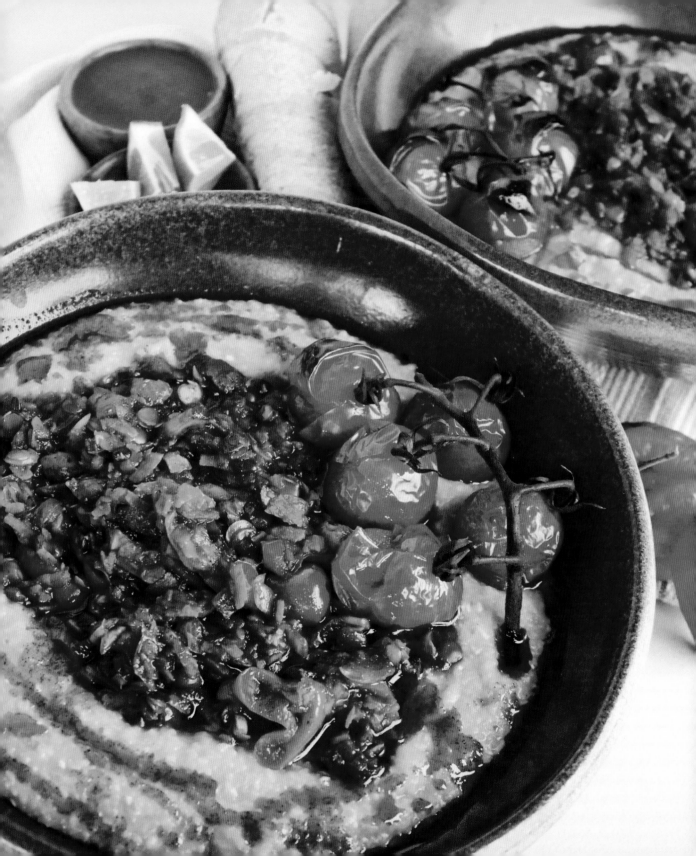

POLENTA WITH SPICY TOMATO CHORIZO

This is Mexican comfort food that's off the beaten path of typical Mexican cuisine. Corn is used in so many different ways down south, which is why I wanted to highlight polenta in this recipe. Although I love a good corn tortilla, this is a delicious way to switch things up and is so simple to make! Chorizo is famous for its paprika and spicy flavor—it truly is Mexican soul food. All of this can be beautifully represented in the plant-based world, as you'll soon experience. This dish is healthy Mexican comfort food and is perfect to share on a warm night in.

THE GOODS

POLENTA

3 cups (720 ml) Immune-Boosting Veggie Broth (page 170)

1 tsp salt

1 cup (150 g) cornmeal

½ cup (120 ml) full-fat coconut milk

CHORIZO

1 tsp olive oil

1 medium onion, chopped

2 tsp (10 g) salt, divided

3 cloves garlic, minced

1 tsp paprika

½ tsp ground coriander

½ tsp ground cumin

¼ tsp chipotle powder, plus more as needed

1½ cups (105 g) finely chopped cremini mushrooms

1 small yellow bell pepper, finely chopped

1 small sweet potato, shredded

1 tbsp (15 ml) agave nectar

¼ cup (40 g) lentils, rinsed

¼ cup (40 g) cherry tomatoes, thinly sliced

2 cups (480 ml) Immune-Boosting Veggie Broth (page 170), divided

GARNISHES

10 cherry tomatoes (preferably on the vine), broiled until blistered

Chili oil

Lime wedges

THE METHOD

First, get your polenta going. In a small saucepan over medium heat, combine the broth and salt. Once the broth is boiling, add the cornmeal while stirring it constantly with a spatula. Reduce the heat to medium-low and cook the polenta for 15 minutes, stirring it every minute or so. Pour in the milk and cook the polenta for 5 to 10 minutes, stirring it every so often, until it is thick and smooth. Cover the polenta and keep it warm while you make the chorizo.

To make the chorizo, heat the oil in a large sauté pan over medium heat. Add in the onion and 1 teaspoon of the salt. Cook the onion for 2 minutes, stirring it frequently. Next, toss in the garlic and cook the mixture for 30 seconds, stirring it occasionally. You'll be stirring both the polenta and the chorizo at the same time, so don't walk away quite yet!

Add the paprika, coriander, cumin and chipotle powder. Toast the spices with the onion and garlic for 30 seconds. Toss in the mushrooms, bell pepper, sweet potato and agave. Cook down the vegetables for 5 minutes. Add the lentils, cherry tomatoes and 1 cup (240 ml) of the broth. Cover the pan and cook the mixture for 10 minutes. Uncover the pan and add the remaining 1 cup (240 ml) of broth. Cook the chorizo, uncovered, for 10 minutes, until the broth is absorbed and the sweet potato is tender.

Taste your chorizo for doneness—the lentils should be tender—and your desired level of spiciness; if you want the chorizo to be spicier, add more chipotle powder. Add the remaining 1 teaspoon of salt, adjusting the amount to your taste if needed. Grab three serving bowls and divide the polenta among them. Top the polenta with the chorizo, blistered cherry tomatoes, chili oil and lime wedges. Serve the polenta and chorizo immediately.

Makes 3 servings

SEARED SWEET POTATO FLAUTAS AND AVOCADO SALSA VERDE

Flautas, taquitos and rolled tacos are all in the same family and all share a special place in my heart. Flautas come in a bigger portion size, which means they hit the spot when you're hungry. The filling on these guys is a little bit of everything I love about vegan Mexican food: The raw ground walnuts add an amazing meaty texture and pair perfectly with the spices and sweetness of the sweet potatoes. This will become one of your go-to recipes when you're having friends over for margaritas.

THE GOODS

AVOCADO SALSA VERDE

8 medium tomatillos, peeled and cut in half

1 cup (40 g) fresh cilantro leaves and stems

2 scallions, coarsely chopped

1 medium jalapeño pepper, deseeded

3 cloves garlic, peeled

3 tbsp (45 ml) fresh lime juice

1 medium avocado, peeled

1 tsp salt

FLAUTAS

3 cups (426 g) coarsely chopped sweet potatoes

1 (15-oz [425-g]) can pinto beans, drained and rinsed

½ cup (50 g) ground walnuts

1 tsp salt

¼ tsp black pepper

½ tsp granulated garlic

½ tsp ground coriander

½ tsp smoked paprika

¼ tsp chipotle powder

10 corn tortillas

2 tbsp (30 ml) avocado oil

GARNISHES

Cashew Cream (page 173)

Finely chopped fresh cilantro

Thinly sliced hot pepper

Lime wedges

THE METHOD

Make the salsa verde first. In a blender, combine the tomatillos, cilantro, scallions, jalapeño, garlic, lime juice, avocado and salt. Pulse the ingredients 10 to 15 times, until smooth, then transfer the salsa to a bowl and set aside.

Next, make the flautas. Fill a medium pot with a small amount of water and insert a steamer basket. Place the sweet potatoes in the basket. Set the pot over medium-low heat, cover the pot and bring the water to a boil. Steam the sweet potatoes for about 10 minutes, until they are fork-tender. Drain the sweet potatoes and transfer them to a large bowl. Add the beans, walnuts, salt, black pepper, granulated garlic, coriander, smoked paprika and chipotle powder. Mash everything together with a fork until well combined and all the spices are evenly incorporated. Set aside.

In a dry small sauté pan or on a flat top grill over medium heat, cook your tortillas for 30 seconds on each side, just until they are warm. Transfer each cooked tortilla to a tortilla warmer or a bowl covered with a kitchen towel, so they can steam and soften before you roll them. Don't skip this step or your tortillas might break as you try to roll them.

Scoop about ½ cup (120 g) of the filling and create a line with it in the middle of a tortilla. Roll the tortilla over the mixture until you've created a rolled taco. Repeat with the remaining filling and tortillas. Heat your oil in a large sauté pan over medium-high heat. Add your flautas to the pan with the seam side down. This will help the flautas stay together. Cook them for 3 to 5 minutes, turning them as needed to ensure that they cook evenly, until they are golden brown and crispy on all sides.

Garnish the flautas with the Cashew Cream, cilantro, hot pepper slices and lime wedges, and serve them with the avocado salsa verde. Try picking these up and eating them with your fingers rather than a fork for a fun take on dinner.

Makes 10 flautas and 2 cups (480 ml) of salsa

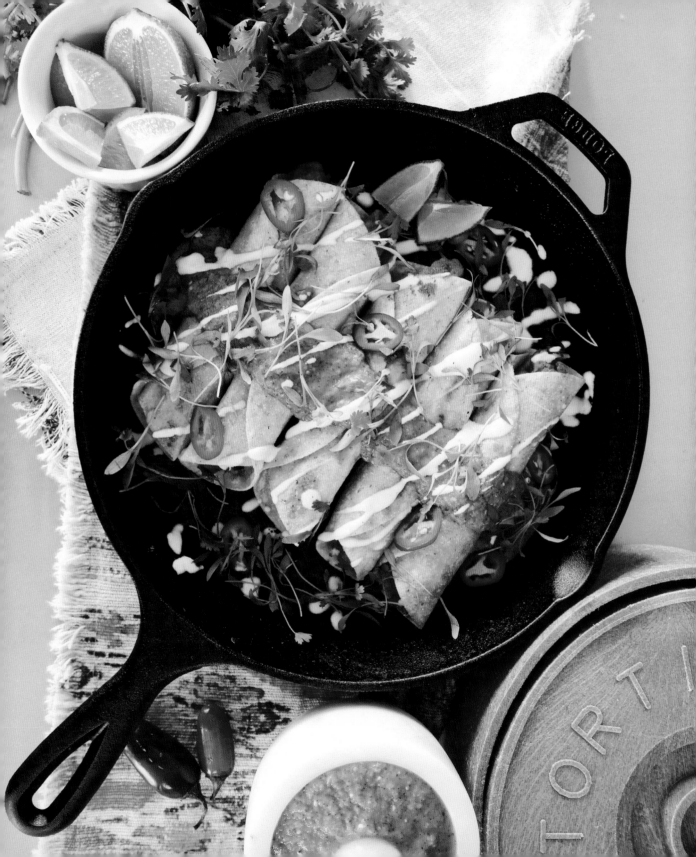

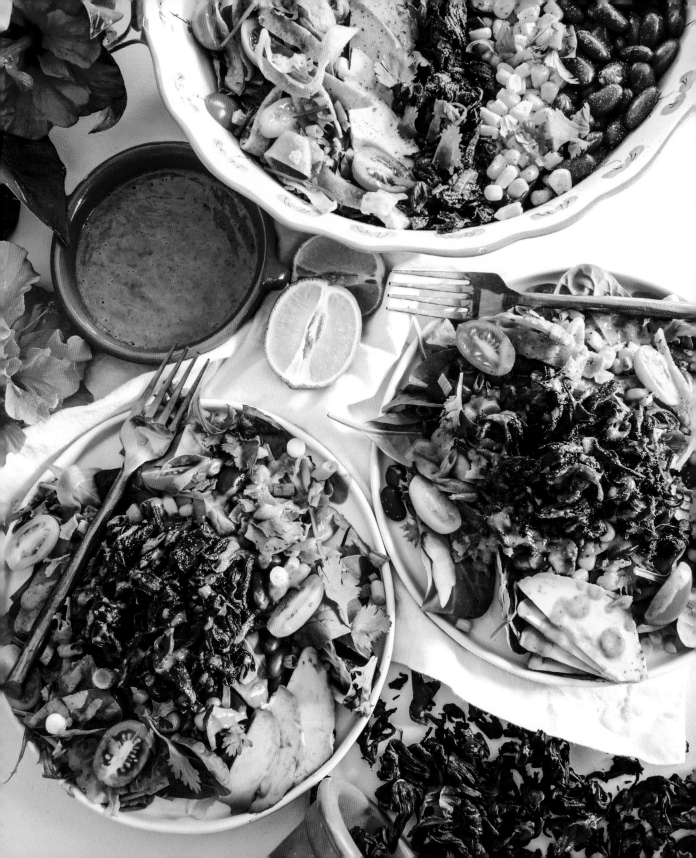

HIBISCUS TACO SALAD

Hibiscus is known for symbolizing youth, beauty and abundance, as well as for its wealth of antioxidants, its ability to lower blood pressure and its support of the liver. Dried hibiscus flowers make for the most amazing tea and—wait for it—vegan meat! The flavor and texture is incredibly similar to shredded beef—you almost won't believe it was once a flower. Once you get the hang of cooking hibiscus flowers in this way, you can make it Asian-inspired, Moroccan-inspired and, most importantly, Mexican-inspired for the best taco salad you've ever had!

THE GOODS

HIBISCUS MEAT

6 cups (1.4 L) water

2 cups (90 g) dried hibiscus flowers

3¼ cups (780 ml) Immune-Boosting Veggie Broth (page 170), divided

1 tbsp (15 ml) liquid aminos

1 tbsp (15 ml) olive oil

½ medium red onion, thinly sliced

½ tsp salt, plus more as needed

1 tsp ground coriander

1 tbsp (15 ml) agave nectar

1 tsp granulated garlic

1 tsp Mexican hot sauce of choice

TANGY AVOCADO DRESSING

½ medium avocado, peeled

½ cup (20 g) fresh cilantro leaves

¼ cup (60 ml) fresh lime juice

2 tbsp (30 ml) agave nectar

½ tsp salt

½ tsp black pepper

½ cup (120 ml) water

1 tbsp (15 ml) white wine vinegar

SALAD

1 tbsp (15 ml) olive oil

4 to 5 corn tortillas, thinly sliced

10 oz (283 g) spring salad mix

1 cup (130 g) corn kernels

1½ cups (230 g) drained and rinsed dark red kidney beans

½ medium avocado, thinly sliced

¼ cup (25 g) diced scallions

½ cup (75 g) cherry tomatoes, cut in half

THE METHOD

In a medium saucepan over high heat, combine the water and hibiscus flowers. Bring the water and hibiscus to a boil, and cook it for 10 minutes. Drain the hibiscus and save the water for a later time—it makes really strong and delicious hibiscus tea. Place the hibiscus back in the empty saucepan. Add 3 cups (720 ml) of the broth and the liquid aminos. Bring the mixture to a boil over high heat, and cook the hibiscus for 15 minutes. Drain the hibiscus, rinse with cold water and squeeze out excess water with your hands. Set the hibiscus aside.

Heat the oil in a large sauté pan over medium-high heat. Add the onion and salt. Cook the onion for 2 to 3 minutes. Add the hibiscus and cook it for 2 minutes, stirring it frequently. Slowly stir in the coriander, agave, additional salt and granulated garlic. Add the remaining ¼ cup (60 ml) of broth to deglaze the bottom of the pan. Now add the hot sauce and cook the mixture for 3 to 4 minutes, stirring it frequently, until the liquid has evaporated and the hibiscus is slightly crispy yet tender. Remove the pan from the heat and set it aside.

Next, make the tangy avocado dressing. In a high-powered blender, combine the avocado, cilantro, lime juice, agave, salt, black pepper, water and vinegar. Blend the ingredients on high speed for 30 seconds, or until the dressing is smooth. Set aside.

Next, make the fried tortilla strips by heating the oil in a medium sauté pan over medium-high heat. Fry the tortilla strips for 3 to 5 minutes, tossing them as they cook, until they are crispy. Set aside.

To assemble the salad, in a large serving bowl or individual serving plates, layer the spring salad mix, corn, beans, tortilla strips, avocado, scallions, cherry tomatoes and hibiscus meat. Drizzle the top of the salad with the tangy avocado dressing and serve immediately.

BAI'S TIP: *You can find dried hibiscus at most Mexican markets or online. Even if it's not at the closest grocery store, don't let that deter you from making this recipe—it's so worth it!*

Makes 5 servings

SPICY MAPLE SLOW COOKER CHILI

When you're vegan, chili is something you can actually live off of. The main vegan staples are beans, rice and quinoa, and although it may seem boring at first, the options between legumes and grains are actually endless. Fiber, plant-based protein and complex carbs play a crucial role in our overall health and an equally crucial role in variety in vegan recipes. Chili is as classic as it gets, with so many flavors and opportunities to sneak in veggies and nutrients. Like any good soup, this recipe will get better with time—and since it's a slow cooker recipe, it's truly a fuss-free twist on a classic and so dang good.

THE GOODS

1 (15-oz [425-g]) can black beans, drained and rinsed

1 (15-oz [425-g]) can great northern beans, drained and rinsed

1 (15-oz [425-g]) can pinto beans, drained and rinsed

1 (8-oz [227-g]) package cremini mushrooms, quartered

2 small sweet potatoes, shredded

1 large tomato, diced

½ cup (100 g) quinoa

1 medium serrano pepper, deseeded

1 large carrot, diced

4 cloves garlic, thinly sliced

1 medium yellow onion, diced

1 large orange bell pepper, diced

2 large ribs celery, diced

1 tsp ground cumin

1 tsp ground coriander

1 tsp salt, plus more as needed

1 tsp black pepper

2 tsp (6 g) smoked paprika

1 tbsp (3 g) finely chopped fresh oregano

1 tbsp (15 ml) pure maple syrup

4 cups (960 ml) Immune-Boosting Veggie Broth (page 170)

Toppings of your choice (see Bai's Tip)

THE METHOD

In a 5- to 7-quart (5- to 7-L) slow cooker, combine the black beans, great northern beans, pinto beans, mushrooms, sweet potatoes, tomato, quinoa, serrano pepper, carrot, garlic, onion, bell pepper, celery, cumin, coriander, salt, black pepper, smoked paprika, oregano, maple syrup and broth. Mix the ingredients well, cover the slow cooker and cook the chili on high for 6 to 8 hours, until the chili is thick and the sweet potatoes and carrot are soft.

Taste the chili for salt and add more if needed. Divide the chili among six bowls and serve it with any toppings you'd like.

BAI'S TIP: The sky's the limit on what you can top this chili with! My favorites as shown in the photo are: Cashew Cream (page 173), thinly sliced tortillas, sliced scallions, lime wedges, shredded vegan cheese, chopped fresh cilantro, hot sauce, sliced radish and chopped or sliced avocado.

Makes 6 servings

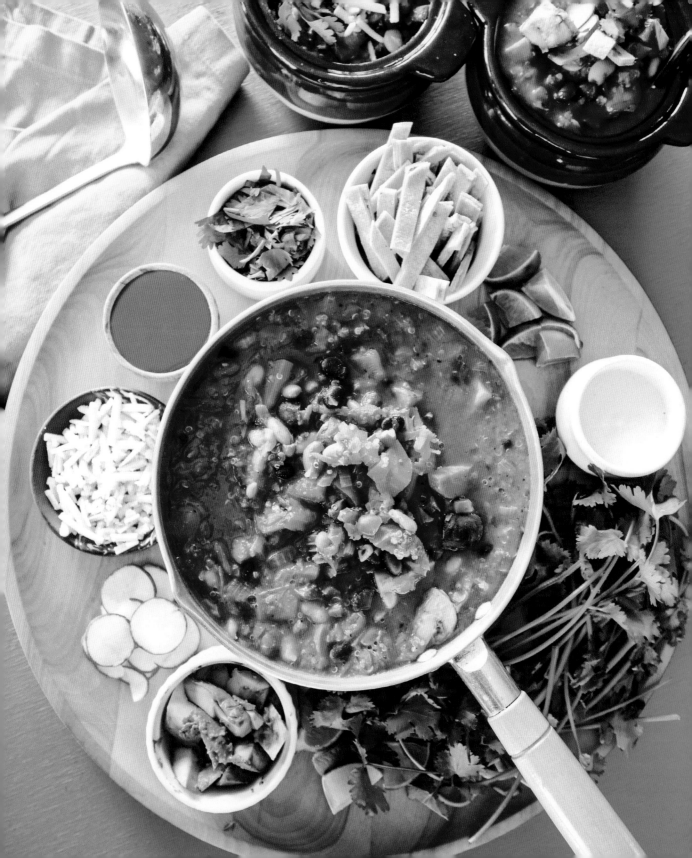

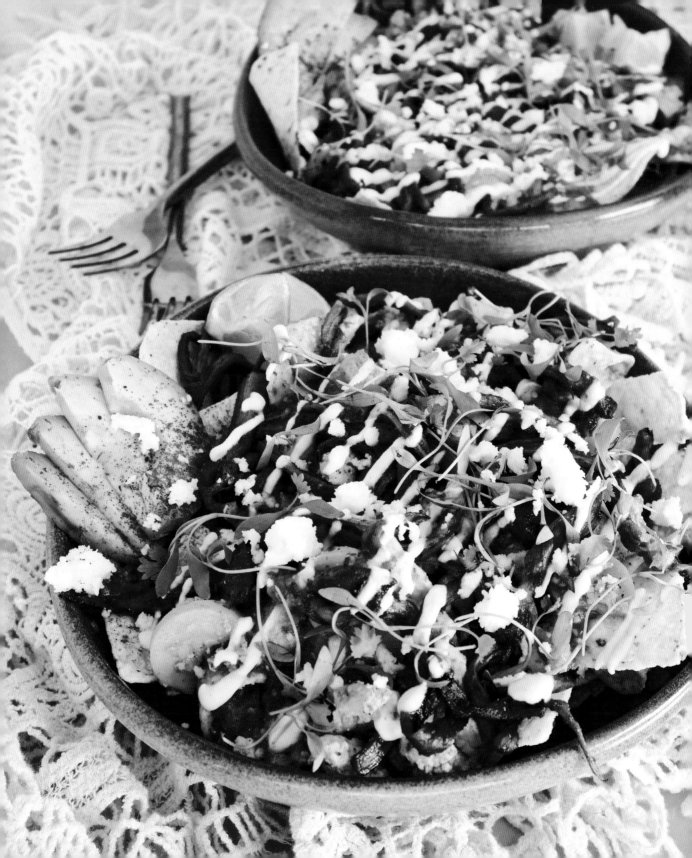

CHILAQUILES

Chilaquiles is my most favorite Mexican breakfast ever. Yes, ever! This dish is classic, and it's always served a little differently depending on where in Mexico you are. The gist of chilaquiles is chips or fried tortillas, smothered in a verde or rojo salsa, that are traditionally served with eggs, cheese and sour cream. To veganize this dish, I'll show you how to make an easy tofu scramble that tastes exactly like eggs—with the added benefit that it's higher in protein with none of the cholesterol of eggs. This is the perfect brunch or holiday breakfast, or it's just my go-to when I need to get transported back to Mexico.

THE GOODS

SALSA VERDE

2½ cups (600 ml) Immune-Boosting Veggie Broth (page 170), divided

1 small yellow onion, thinly sliced

1 tsp salt, divided

8 medium tomatillos, quartered

1 medium jalapeño pepper, deseeded and finely chopped

1 (4-oz [113-g]) can diced green chilies, undrained

3 cloves garlic, finely chopped

¼ tsp ground cumin

¼ tsp ground coriander

½ cup (20 g) fresh cilantro leaves, minced

TOFU SCRAMBLE

1 tsp olive oil

1 medium shallot, thinly sliced

Pinch plus ½ tsp Himalayan pink salt, divided

1 (14-oz [397-g]) block firm tofu, drained

½ tsp ground turmeric

½ tsp black salt

1 yellow summer squash, chopped

CHILAQUILES

6 cups (156 g) tortilla chips

Carnitas Mushrooms (page 66; optional)

1 medium avocado, thinly sliced

Cashew Cream (page 173; optional)

¼ cup (6 g) micro greens

THE METHOD

First, make the salsa verde. In a medium saucepan over medium-high heat, combine ¼ cup (60 ml) of the broth, onion and ½ teaspoon of the salt. Stir the ingredients together and cook the onion for 2 minutes, until it starts to soften. Add the tomatillos, jalapeño, green chilies and their juice, garlic, cumin, coriander, remaining 2¼ cups (540 ml) of broth and remaining ½ teaspoon of salt. Reduce the heat to medium-low, cover the saucepan and cook the salsa for 15 minutes. Stir in the cilantro, then carefully transfer the salsa to a blender and blend it until it is smooth. This salsa should be a bit runny and not super thick. Keep it warm by pouring it back in your saucepan and setting it over low heat until everything else is ready. If you have extra salsa at the end, store it in the fridge for a great appetizer with chips.

While your sauce is cookin', make the tofu scramble. Heat the oil in a medium sauté pan over medium-high heat. Add the shallot and pinch of Himalayan pink salt. Cook the shallot for 2 minutes, then use your hands to crumble the block of tofu into tiny pieces over the pan—think feta cheese while you're crumbling the tofu. Add the turmeric and black salt, reduce the heat to medium and cook the tofu for 3 to 5 minutes. Toss in the squash and the remaining ½ teaspoon of Himalayan pink salt. Mix everything together and cook the tofu scramble for 2 minutes, until the squash has started to soften. Remove the pan from the heat, cover it and set it aside.

To assemble the chilaquiles, grab two serving bowls. Divide the chips between both bowls. Pour half of the salsa verde over each serving of chips. We want to smother these chips with salsa-verde love, so don't be shy! Top each bowl with half of the tofu scramble and Carnitas Mushrooms (if using). Garnish each serving with half of the avocado slices, a drizzle of the Cashew Cream (if using) and half of the micro greens. Serve the chilaquiles immediately.

Makes 2 servings

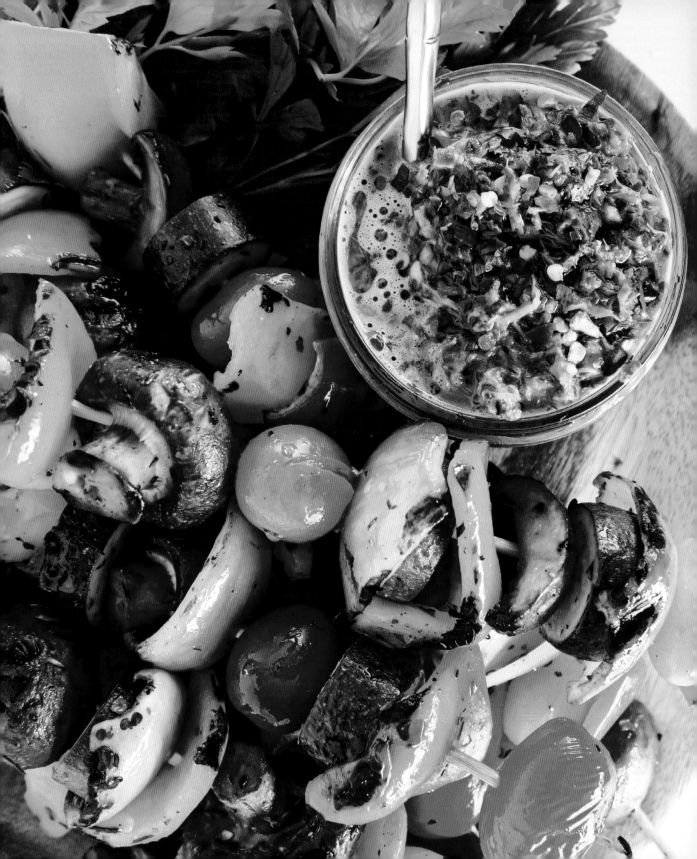

QUICK AND *Healthy*

This chapter is for all you working professionals and parents out there. Actually, this section is also for the college students, the grandparents, the athletes and everyone in between. We all need quick, nutrient-dense recipes to carry us through the day, the week, the month and our entire lives that are affordable and made with easy-to-find ingredients.

Nutrient-dense food is food that doesn't have empty calories or calories that contain hydrogenated oils, preservatives, fillers, chemicals and refined sweeteners like high-fructose corn syrup. Essentially, you're getting the most out of your calories by cooking with and eating food that's filled with nutrients and, in turn, a whole lot of flavor. There's a common misconception that the more vibrant something is, the weirder it tastes—actually, vibrancy in our produce means big and bright flavor. We're getting away from the beige-food rut and moving toward ingredients that allow us to taste the rainbow our amazing planet and hardworking farmers have to offer us.

When eating and cooking the rainbow, you're getting a diversity of plants and foods in your daily diet, which is like taking a multivitamin but way more exciting. The greater diversity of plants you eat, the more you're taking care of different parts of your body. For example, carrots are good for your eyes, while beets help support brain health, while strawberries are good for heart health . . . Starting to catch on? Instead of listing out every fruit, veggie, grain, nut and legume, the idea here is that the more diversely you eat, the more you are helping heal and support your whole body.

I cooked food for the majority of my life with only one thing on my mind: flavor. During that time, I loved to eat and I loved to cook, but my connection to the food was surface level. I didn't have a connection to the earth and my own body, which I learned are crucial parts of being truly connected to food. The surface-level pleasure food I was cooking was actually feeding my endometriosis and causing me so much suffering on the inside for only a few moments of enjoyment. Food either fights disease or feeds it, and I learned the hard way which side I wanted to be on.

What I realized is that you don't have to compromise flavor for nutrients—you just have to rethink how you're going about it! An open mind is helpful while beginning this process, but I assure you it's life changing. This entire book is packed to the brim with nutrient-dense recipes, but this chapter in particular has recipes that are simple to make and very veggie-forward. If you are someone who "doesn't like" veggies—or if you are cooking for someone who is wary of veggies—I challenge you to think differently and look at your taste buds as a muscle you have to flex. Get cookin' with this chapter, flex those muscles, activate your cravings and taste the rainbow!

THIRTY-MINUTE MARINARA AND GARLICKY SPAGHETTI SQUASH

Everyone needs a weeknight meal that's easy to throw together, takes minimal ingredients, nourishes the body and hits those comfort-food spots after a long day. This recipe meets all those needs. This marinara will change the way you think about making marinara from scratch. Don't get me wrong, I love a good four-hour marinara, but in the real world, nobody has time for that. All you need is some fresh ingredients and 30 minutes for a marinara that you don't even have to stir. Top this dish with Walnut Parm (page 161) and you've got yourself a winner.

THE GOODS

MARINARA

3 lb (1.4 kg) heirloom tomatoes, destemmed (beefsteak tomatoes work great too)

1 medium yellow onion, thinly sliced

3 cloves garlic, peeled

2 tbsp (30 ml) olive oil

1 tsp salt

1 tsp black pepper

GARLICKY SPAGHETTI SQUASH

1 medium spaghetti squash, cut in half lengthwise and deseeded

2 tbsp (30 ml) olive oil

½ tsp salt

½ tsp black pepper

1 tsp granulated garlic

½ tsp red pepper flakes

1 tsp finely chopped fresh basil

Walnut Parm (page 161), as needed

THE METHOD

First, make the marinara. Preheat your oven to 375°F (191°C). Cut the tomatoes into quarters. On a large baking sheet, arrange the tomatoes, onion and garlic. Add the oil, salt and black pepper. Using your hands, toss the vegetables in the oil and seasonings until the tomatoes are covered in the seasonings. Set the baking sheet aside.

Now it's time to prepare the garlicky spaghetti squash. On a separate large baking sheet, arrange the squash halves face up and add the oil, salt, black pepper and granulated garlic. Rub the oil and spices on the squash halves until they are covered on the inside. Turn the squash halves face down on the baking sheet.

Pop both the marinara vegetables and the squash into oven and roast them for 25 minutes.

After 25 minutes, remove the marinara vegetables from the oven, and roast the squash for another 15 minutes. While the squash is roasting, transfer the marinara vegetables and any accumulated juices to a blender. You can pulse the blender to create a chunky marinara, or you can puree it so it's smooth—up to you!

You'll know your squash is done when you press the outside of it with a wooden spoon and it's soft—the spoon will press into the squash a little. Pull your squash from the oven, let it cool for 3 to 5 minutes and then flip each half over. Shred the squash with a fork to create "spaghetti." Divide the squash between three serving bowls. Top the squash with the marinara, red pepper flakes, basil and Walnut Parm.

BAI'S TIP: If you're looking to add some protein to this, you can add cooked lentils to your sauce or some garbanzo beans that have been sautéed in a little olive oil and salt. Both work great!

Makes 3 servings

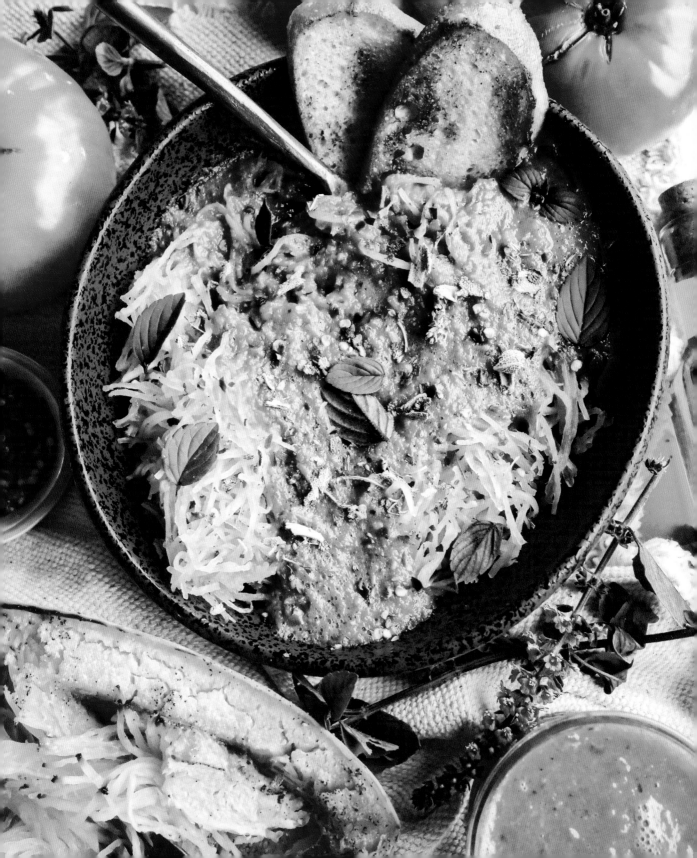

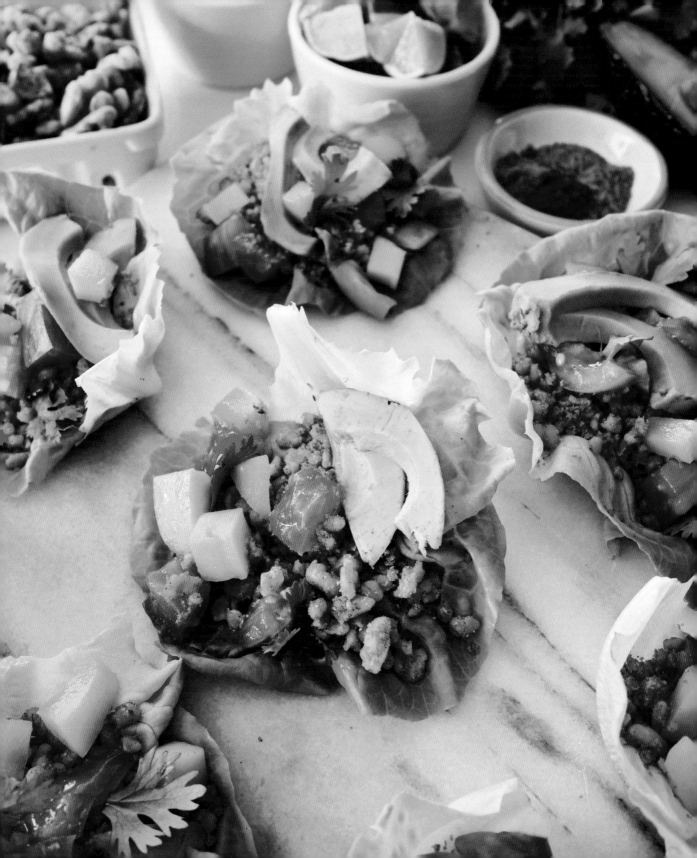

RAW WALNUT LETTUCE TACOS

I know the title of this recipe alone may make you feel that it's way outside your comfort zone. You may be thinking, "Okay, Bai, I'm getting down with this plant-based stuff, but raw tacos with walnuts as meat? Seems wild," and I'm here to tell you that walnut meat is not only thought provoking but also a delicious game changer in the nut aisle. This completely raw dish takes only ten minutes to throw together. It's rich in protein, nutrients and flavor. You can always use the walnut meat as a protein-dense topper for a taco salad too. I love having these tacos on deck when I'm on a cleanse or just wanting to eat mindfully for my body. Light, fresh, filling and crazy good!

THE GOODS

WALNUT MEAT

2 cups (230 g) raw walnuts

½ tsp ground cumin

½ tsp ground coriander

½ tsp garlic powder

1 tsp salt

½ tsp paprika

½ tsp black pepper

1 tbsp (15 ml) melted coconut oil (optional)

TACOS

12 leaves butter lettuce

1 medium mango, peeled and diced

1 medium tomato, diced

2 medium avocados, thinly sliced

¼ cup (10 g) fresh cilantro leaves

Hot sauce of choice, as needed

1 medium lime, cut in half

THE METHOD

To make the walnut meat, combine the walnuts, cumin, coriander, garlic powder, salt, paprika, black pepper and oil (if using) in a blender or food processor. Pulse the ingredients about ten times. We don't want the walnuts to turn to powder—the meat should be chunky. Set the walnut meat aside.

Assemble your tacos by grabbing a serving platter and placing your lettuce leaves on the platter. Put 2 to 3 tablespoons (30 to 45 g) of your walnut meat in each taco. You may have some extra, and that's okay—save it for a rainy day or more tacos! Next, add a few mango pieces, tomato pieces, avocado slices, cilantro leaves and dashes of hot sauce to each taco. Finish them by squeezing the lime over the platter of tacos. Serve the tacos immediately.

BAI'S TIP: *Use this concept for walnut meat as a ground beef substitute in Italian recipes like Bolognese and lasagna. Just season the meat with basil, garlic and salt instead of Mexican seasonings!*

Makes 12 tacos

KALE CAESAR SALAD

Although a Caesar salad is a salad, typically there isn't anything too healthy about it other than the fact that there's some lettuce serving as a vehicle for raw egg yolk, lots of oil, cheese and a ton of salt! When reading through these ingredients, you might think, "There's no way this is going to compare." Well, it does—and it's damn good too! With tons of Caesar salad flavor and plant protein as the main element in the dressing, this recipe will change how you look at this iconic dish.

THE GOODS

SALAD

1 large cauliflower, cut into florets

1 (15-oz [425-g]) can garbanzo beans, drained and rinsed

3 cloves garlic

2 tbsp (30 ml) olive oil, divided

1 tsp garlic powder

1 tsp salt

½ tsp black pepper

1 tbsp (3 g) dried basil

½ tsp paprika

1 tbsp (15 ml) pure maple syrup

1 large bunch kale, destemmed and thinly sliced

1 medium avocado, thickly sliced

CROUTONS

3 slices ciabatta bread, cubed

1 tbsp (15 ml) olive oil

½ tsp granulated garlic

¼ tsp salt

¼ tsp black pepper

DRESSING

1 cup (150 g) drained and rinsed garbanzo beans

1 tbsp (15 g) Dijon mustard

1 tbsp (15 g) capers with brine

1 tsp salt

1 tsp granulated garlic

1 tsp black pepper

1 tbsp (5 g) nutritional yeast

1 tbsp (15 g) tahini

3 tbsp (45 ml) fresh lemon juice

1 cup (240 ml) water

THE METHOD

To make the salad, preheat your oven to 375°F (191°C). On a large baking sheet, toss together your cauliflower florets, beans and garlic. Drizzle 1 tablespoon (15 ml) of the oil over the cauliflower mixture and top the mixture with the garlic powder, salt, black pepper, basil, paprika and maple syrup. Toss the mixture with your hands to thoroughly combine the ingredients. Roast the mixture for 20 minutes, until the cauliflower is golden brown and the beans are slightly crispy.

While the veggies are roasting, make the croutons. Grab a medium baking sheet and toss together the bread cubes, oil, granulated garlic, salt and black pepper. Place the croutons in the oven and toast them during the last 5 minutes of the veggies' roasting time, until the croutons are crispy on the outside and slightly soft on the inside. Remove both baking sheets at the same time.

To make the dressing, combine 1 cup (100 g) of the roasted cauliflower florets, roasted garlic, garbanzo beans, mustard, capers and their brine, salt, granulated garlic, black pepper, nutritional yeast, tahini, lemon juice and water in a blender. Blend the ingredients for 30 seconds, until the dressing is smooth. Set the dressing aside.

Now it's time to make your salads. Place the kale in a large bowl and drizzle the remaining 1 tablespoon (15 ml) of oil over it. Massage the kale with your hands for about 2 minutes, until its volume has reduced by about one-third. Divide your kale among three bowls, then top it with the roasted veggies and beans, croutons, avocado slices and some of the dressing.

BAI'S TIP: Turn this recipe into a Caesar wrap by wrapping the contents for one bowl into a large tortilla. It's the perfect on-the-go salad!

Makes 3 servings

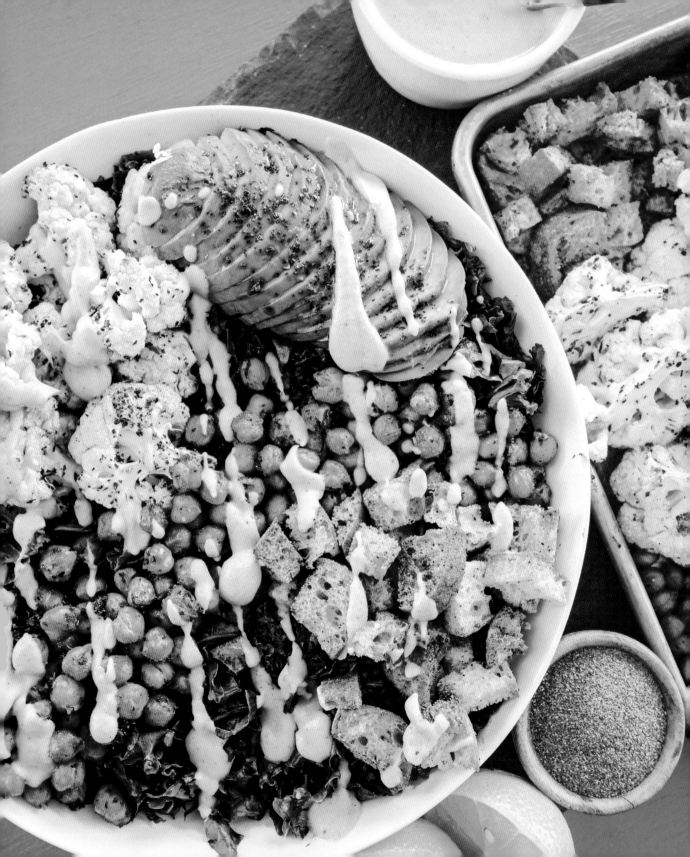

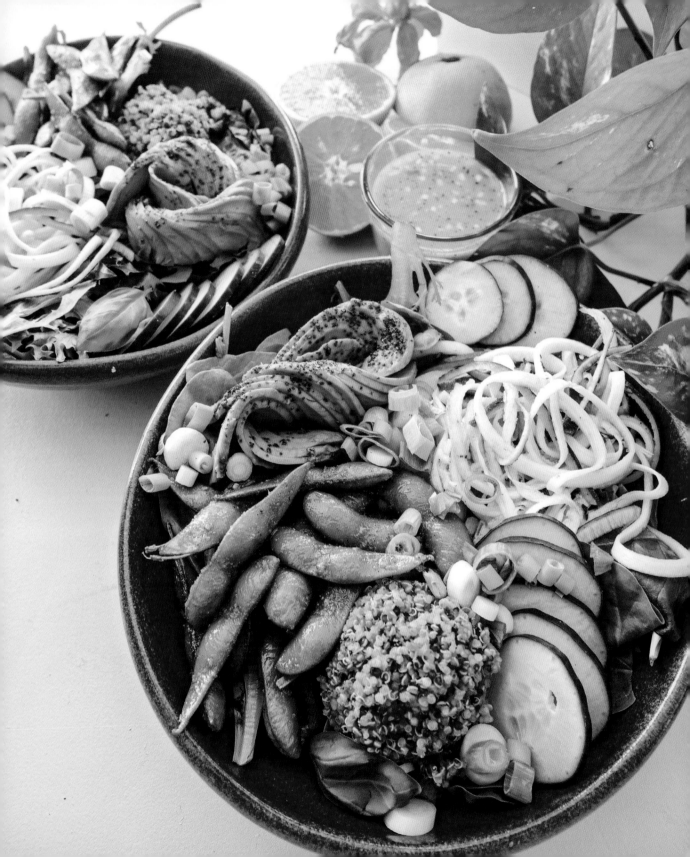

THE GARDEN BOWL WITH CITRUS-SHALLOT DRESSING

This dish is as quick and healthy as it gets. I always measure if I'm on track to my health goals by how many greens I've had in one day. Eating one of these bowls puts you in the winner's circle for daily greens. A meal-prep hack I started using years ago is to always make sure I have some sort of high-protein grain or legume prepped and ready to go in my fridge. Quinoa, lentils and garbanzo beans all store amazingly well in the fridge and are good cold on salads just like this one. I chose quinoa for this bowl, but any of those three would work great in this recipe. Make your meal-prep plan, and be sure to put this recipe on there. Your skin will glow, your digestion will be smooth and your overall energy will be high after diving into this bowl of green goodness.

THE GOODS

BOWLS

1 tbsp (15 ml) olive oil

1 cup (100 g) fresh or thawed frozen edamame pods

¼ tsp salt

¼ tsp granulated garlic

4 packed cups (400 g) baby spinach

1 cup (100 g) raw zucchini noodles

½ cup (120 g) cooked quinoa

1 medium avocado, thinly sliced

¼ medium cucumber, thinly sliced

¼ cup (30 g) thinly sliced scallions

CITRUS-SHALLOT DRESSING

¼ cup (60 ml) fresh orange juice

1 tbsp (15 ml) fresh lemon juice

1 tbsp (15 ml) olive oil

¼ tsp salt, plus more as needed

¼ tsp black pepper

1 tbsp (10 g) minced shallots

1 tbsp (15 ml) white wine vinegar

THE METHOD

First, prepare the bowls. Heat the oil in a large sauté pan over medium-high heat. Add the edamame pods, salt and granulated garlic. Sauté the edamame for 3 minutes, stirring the pods frequently, until the garlic is golden brown and the pods are cooked but not mushy. Remove the pan from the heat and set it aside.

Now make the citrus-shallot dressing. In a 16-ounce (454-g) Mason jar, combine the orange juice, lemon juice, oil, salt, black pepper, minced shallots and vinegar. Top the jar with its lid, close the lid tightly and shake what your mama gave ya to create the dressing. Taste the dressing for saltiness with a piece of spinach, and add more salt if needed. Set the dressing aside.

Assemble your bowls by grabbing two shallow serving bowls. In each bowl, place half of the spinach, zucchini noodles, quinoa, avocado, cooked edamame, cucumber and sliced scallions. Drizzle the dressing over the top and serve the bowls immediately.

BAI'S TIP: Edmame shells are very tough and should not be eaten whole. Make sure to pop the beans out of the pods when eating!

Makes 2 servings

MEDITERRANEAN VEGGIE SKEWERS WITH CHIMICHURRI

Just because we're cookin' with plants doesn't mean our grills get the cold shoulder! This recipe is a staple in my house for many reasons! The marinade goes great on anything and I have been swooning over this chimichurri for years. I mean it when I say it's the ultimate, as it's amazing with bread, empanadas and absolutely anything grilled. Bring this to your next family BBQ and you'll have everyone asking you for your secret!

THE GOODS

SKEWERS
9 cremini mushrooms

1 cup (150 g) cherry tomatoes

1 medium zucchini, thickly sliced

1 medium orange bell pepper, chopped into 2" (5-cm) pieces

½ medium red onion, finely chopped

MARINADE
2 tbsp (30 ml) olive oil

1 tbsp (15 g) Dijon mustard

1 tbsp (15 ml) liquid aminos

2 tbsp (30 ml) apple cider vinegar

1 tbsp (15 ml) pure maple syrup

1 tsp salt

½ tsp black pepper

1 tsp dried thyme

1 tsp dried basil

1 tsp dried oregano

CHIMICHURRI
1 medium bunch fresh parsley

1 medium bunch fresh cilantro

1 medium shallot, peeled

½ small jalapeño pepper, deseeded and finely chopped

2 scallions, chopped

2 tbsp (30 ml) fresh lime juice

2 tbsp (30 ml) fresh lemon juice

3 cloves garlic, peeled

3 tbsp (45 ml) red wine vinegar

2 tbsp (30 ml) olive oil

½ tsp salt

¼ cup (60 ml) water

THE METHOD

To prep the skewers, place the mushrooms, tomatoes, zucchini, bell pepper and onion in a large bowl. If any of the mushrooms are very large, cut them in half. Set the bowl aside.

To make the marinade, combine the oil, mustard, liquid aminos, apple cider vinegar, maple syrup, salt, black pepper, thyme, basil and oregano in a small bowl. Mix the ingredients with a spoon until the marinade is smooth.

Pour the marinade over the veggies and toss them until they are fully coated in the marinade. Set the bowl of veggies in the fridge and allow them to marinate for at least 30 minutes, but no longer than 6 hours to avoid soggy veggies.

As the veggies marinate, make the chimichurri. In a high-powered blender, combine the parsley, cilantro, shallot, jalapeño, scallions, lime juice, lemon juice, garlic, red wine vinegar, oil, salt and water. Blend until the chimichurri has some small and chunky pieces but is not fully pureed.

Thread the marinated veggies onto metal or wooden skewers—if you're using wooden skewers, soak them for 5 minutes in water first. Preheat a grill or a grill pan to medium heat. Add the veggie skewers and grill them for 3 to 4 minutes on each side, allowing them to brown and blacken in some spots. Remove the skewers from the heat and serve them on a platter with the chimichurri. This dish makes great leftovers to eat with rice pilaf too!

BAI'S TIP: If you're looking to get a bit of protein on these skewers, 1-inch (2.5-cm) cubes of firm tofu marinate and grill perfectly with this!

Makes 2 to 3 servings

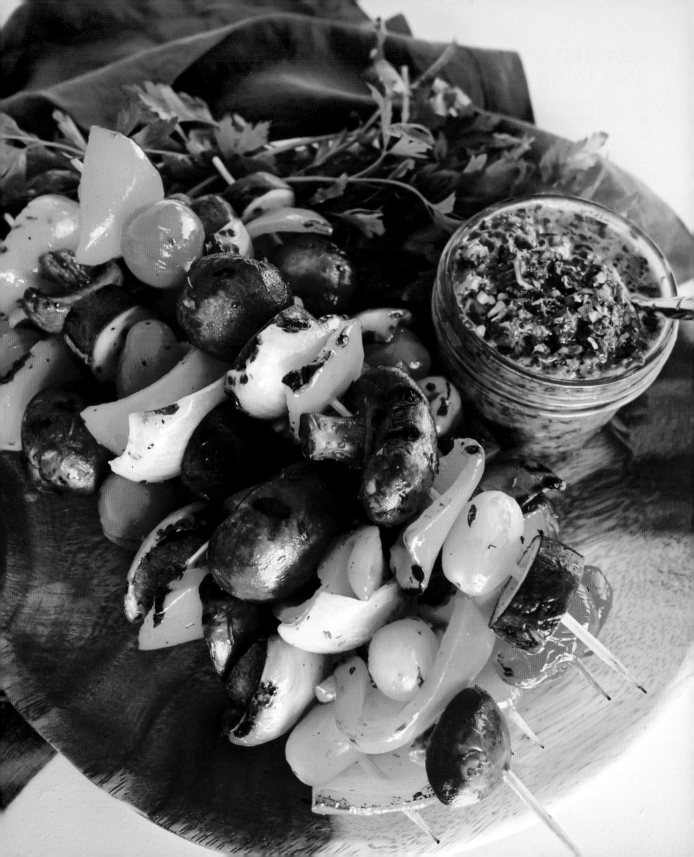

ROASTED SWEET POTATOES WITH CRISPY KALE AND TAHINI DRESSING

This meal is just what you need to fix you up after a long day! I have been making versions of this meal for years, and even before I became vegan, it got me through some long days working multiple jobs and running a business. Sweet potatoes are the ultimate food. They are high in vitamin A and fiber, they're tasty and they help keep our gut healthy! Using our trusted sweet potatoes as a base for this, and then adding the garbanzos, kale chips and tahini dressing? Oh yeah, you're in for a real treat. This is a nutritionally packed meal that's quick to put together and tastes like something you'd get at your favorite neighborhood restaurant!

THE GOODS

SWEET POTATOES AND GARBANZO BEANS

4 large sweet potatoes, cut in half lengthwise

1 (15-oz [425-g]) can garbanzo beans, drained and rinsed

1 tbsp (15 ml) olive oil

1 tsp salt

½ tsp black pepper

2 tbsp (6 g) dried herb blend (I like basil, parsley and tarragon)

1 tsp granulated garlic

1 tbsp (15 ml) pure date or maple syrup

1 large avocado, cubed

KALE CHIPS

1 large bunch kale, destemmed and torn into small pieces

1 tbsp (15 ml) olive oil

½ tsp salt

½ tsp garlic powder

TAHINI DRESSING

3 tbsp (45 g) tahini

1 tbsp (15 ml) pure date or maple syrup

¼ tsp black pepper

¼ tsp salt

¼ cup (60 ml) fresh lemon juice

2 tbsp (30 ml) water

THE METHOD

To make the sweet potatoes and garbanzo beans, preheat the oven to 350°F (177°C). Place the sweet potatoes on a large baking sheet with the sliced side facing upward. Arrange the beans around the sweet potatoes. Cover the potatoes and beans with the oil, salt, black pepper, herb blend, granulated garlic and date syrup. Toss the sweet potatoes and beans with your hands to coat them in the seasoning mixture. Place the potatoes sliced side facing downward on your baking sheet, surrounded by the beans. Roast the sweet potatoes and beans for 30 to 40 minutes, until the sweet potatoes are fork-tender.

Meanwhile, get your kale chips ready to bake. Place the kale on a separate large baking sheet. Cover the kale with the oil, salt and garlic powder. Toss the kale with your hands to coat it in the oil and seasonings.

When the potatoes have about 10 minutes of roasting time left, place the kale chips on the top rack of the oven and bake them for the remaining 10 minutes, until they are crispy but not burned. Both the sweet potatoes and beans and the kale chips should finish at the same time.

As everything is cooking, it's time to make the tahini dressing. In a 16-ounce (454-g) Mason jar, combine the tahini, date syrup, black pepper, salt, lemon juice and water. Secure the jar's lid and shake the jar for 30 seconds, until the dressing ingredients come together. Set the dressing aside.

If the sweet potatoes aren't tender after 30 minutes, pull out the kale and garbanzo beans and cook the sweet potatoes for 10 to 15 minutes more. Once the potatoes are done, let them cool for 3 minutes before serving them.

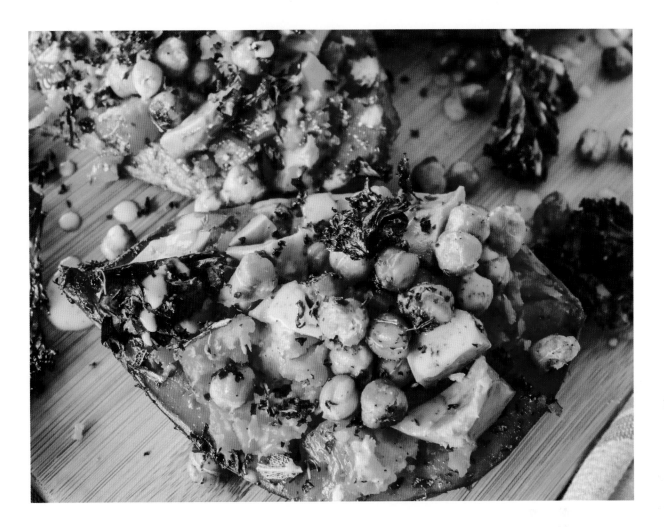

BAI'S TIP: *Organic sweet potatoes have better flavor and cook faster! They are fresher at the supermarket—and because they are not sprayed or genetically modified, they are softer, making them easier to slice and quicker to cook.*

Place two sweet potato halves face up on a plate. Slice each half in half lengthwise, making sure you don't go all the way through the sweet potato. You can push the long sides together to make the sweet potato more of a boat shape. Top each of the sweet potato halves with a handful of the garbanzo beans and one-fourth of the avocado. Lastly, drizzle the dressing over the sweet potato halves to your liking.

Serve the sweet potatoes with side of kale chips, or crumble the kale chips over the top of the potatoes.

Makes 4 servings

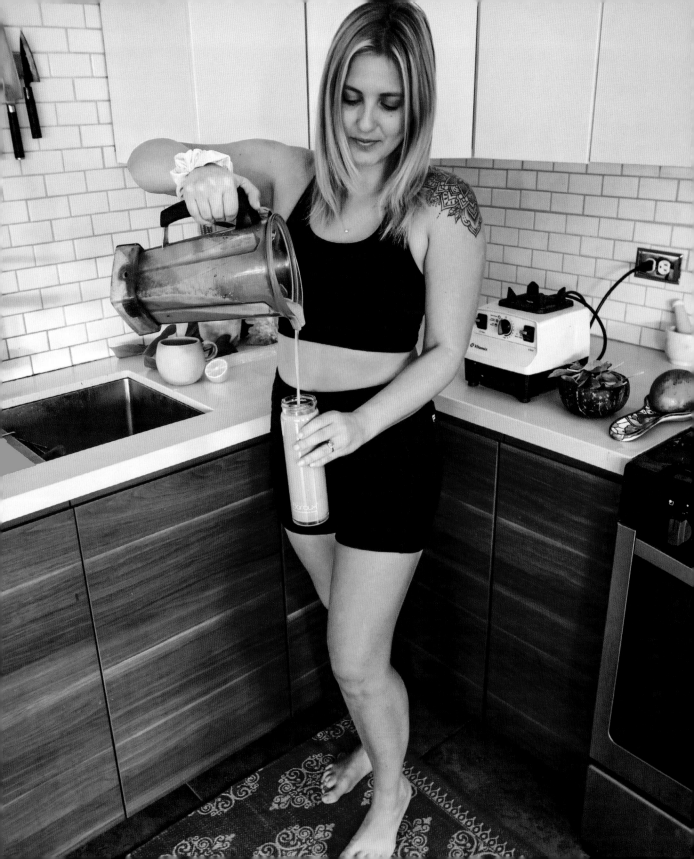

MORNING *Mastery*

If you can master your morning, you can master your entire day. I used to roll my eyes at this concept, and I still don't qualify myself as a morning person. Whether or not you're a morning person won't affect how this morning routine can help you, as it goes way beyond that label. It doesn't matter if you get up at the crack of dawn or 10 a.m., as we all experience our mornings differently.

I used to wake up craving an insane amount of carbs. I'd dive into a bagel with cream cheese, buy a five-dollar latte on my way to work and crash like a five-year-old after a hunger-fueled temper tantrum around 11:30 a.m. I ate like this every day, except for an occasional breakfast treat at one of my favorite neighborhood spots in San Francisco. During this time, I also experienced the most chronic pain from my endometriosis. It's a vicious cycle: waking up feeling like hell, carb-loading to gloss over the problem, getting juiced up on espresso to combat the carbs, crashing from the espresso, eating an unhealthy lunch out of starvation. Rinse and repeat. Every single day.

I know your morning routine is probably not exactly like mine was—although it might be. My point is that at some juncture in our lives, many of us have found ourselves in this vicious cycle, or one like it, more times than we'd like to admit.

My healing journey began when I discovered the power of the green smoothie. Seems pretty simple and ridiculous, but to me it was revolutionary. Instead of going for a bagel or leftover pizza in the morning, I would drink a green smoothie first thing. At first, I tried to go just 7 days starting my day with a green smoothie, as veggies weren't really my thing quite yet. I knew if I could drink something green for 7 days in a row, I'd be set. Pretty soon, 7 days turned into 60 days. And 60 days turned into 4 years. My life began changing because of a simple daily green smoothie, and I started to recognize my body as my own again. I wasn't even close to becoming plant-based yet, but it was the one thing I could do every single day to say to my body, "Hey, I see you, I feel you and I'm trying."

I slowly switched out my vanilla whole-milk latte for a matcha latte with almond milk. My breakfast burrito switched to breakfast tofu tacos with corn tortillas instead of wheat. My chronic dehydration began to dissipate as I realized that if I drank a huge glass of water before my smoothie, I would be a happier person and actually want to show up in this world.

This life-changing journey that started with my mornings has allowed me to develop this collection of recipes, so that I can assist you through your morning routine. I truly believe that if we can change and control what we eat, we can change our lives in positive ways. Mastering your morning means mastering your life, your health and your relationship with yourself.

BAI'S MAPLE MATCHA LATTE

This is it: The juice to start my day. My kick-starter. My rocket fuel. Welcome to the wonderful world of matcha. It's the ultimate pick-me-up in the morning and, in my opinion, way better than coffee. Matcha has less caffeine than coffee, but thanks to the amino acid L-theanine, your body actually processes the caffeine differently. Forget the coffee jitters and afternoon crash—matcha will give you a steady boost while keeping you focused and on your game. Matcha is also less acidic and contains antioxidants, which is a switch your body will love. I pair my matcha with cinnamon, as I feel they are a match made in heaven. When choosing your matcha, check its quality and origin. Farm-direct from Japan, shade-grown, stone-milled matcha is what you're looking for! My favorite brand is Mizuba. Buy as high-quality matcha as your budget allows, because it makes a huge difference in taste and caffeine buzz.

This matcha latte is something I regularly make for guests, my family, my neighbors and myself. I actually have friends that request matcha lattes as a condition to booking their flights! It's that good. This recipe changed my life and the way I look at and feel about my mornings. I hope it can do the same for you.

THE GOODS

1 cup (240 ml) Cashew-Hemp Milk (page 162)

1 cup (240 ml) water

½ tsp ground cinnamon

1 tsp matcha powder

2 tsp (10 ml) pure maple syrup

THE METHOD

In a small pot over low heat, combine the milk and water. Heat the mixture until it begins steaming or is hot to the touch—do not heat it more than this, as the milk may burn.

Transfer the milk and water to a blender. Add the cinnamon, matcha and maple syrup. Blend the ingredients on high speed for at least 2 minutes. This will create an amazing froth to the latte. Pour the latte in your favorite large mug and enjoy it while it's warm.

If you'd like to create the layered effect that's shown in the photo, blend the heated cashew milk alone for 1 minute, then pour it in your mug. After that, combine the water, cinnamon, matcha and maple syrup in the blender, blend the ingredients for 2 minutes and then pour the mixture over the frothy cashew milk to create two layers.

Yields 2 (20-oz [591-ml]) servings

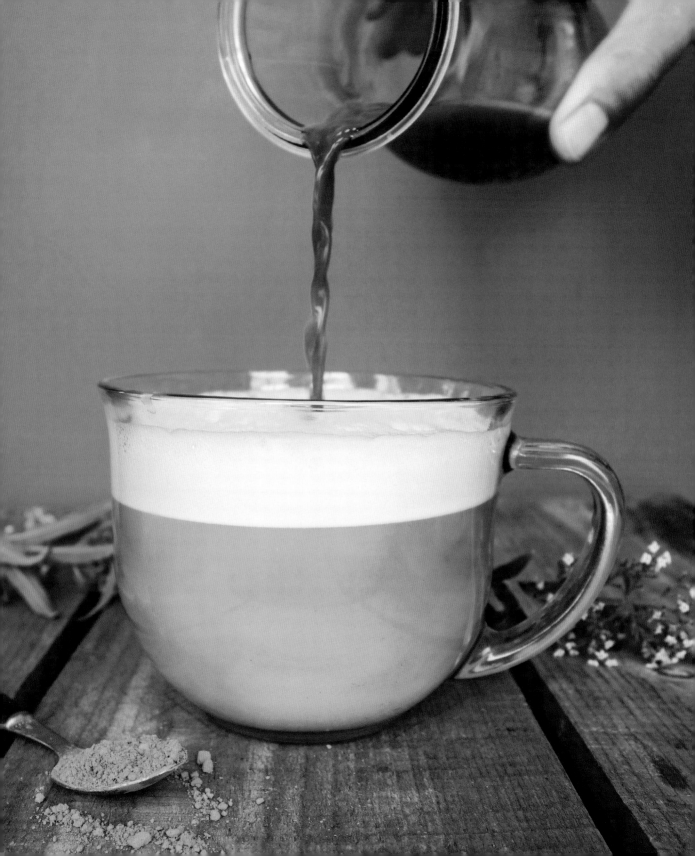

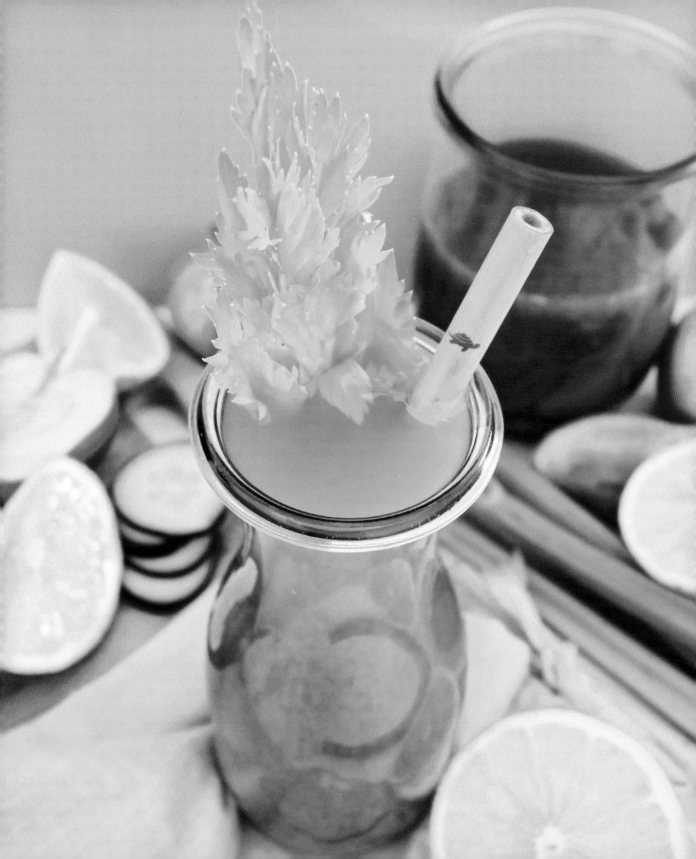

GO-TO GREEN JUICE

Over the years, my daily smoothie has turned into a 32-ounce (946-ml) cold-pressed green juice thanks to the investment in my slow juicer. But don't worry—if you don't have a slow juicer, a high-powered blender can make similar juices. Nothing makes me feel as amazing as a cold-pressed green juice does. It beats a smoothie, coffee and—dare I say it?—even matcha. It's like jumping into a cold pool on a hot day or that energized feeling you get right after an epic yoga class.

Cold-pressed, low-sugar green juices are actually life changing. You get those high-vibrational micronutrients when you drink it on an empty stomach in the morning, and there's nothing quite like it! This particular green juice is my go-to, because I drink it at least five times a week. It's light, easy to drink, great for immune health and, thanks to the cucumbers and romaine, easy on the palate if you're new to eating lots of greens. Parsley is my secret ingredient, as it's incredibly beneficial for your health. This recipe is a sure way to get a concentrated dose of the healing powers of this potent herb. You'll get cleared out and clearheaded in 16 ounces (480 ml), and you'll become a superhero with just 32 ounces (946 ml). This juice will bring you that much closer to mastering your entire day.

THE GOODS

1 large bunch celery, finely chopped

1 large head romaine lettuce, coarsely chopped

3 medium Honeycrisp or Fuji apples, cored and coarsely chopped

1 medium bunch fresh parsley

2 large cucumbers, coarsely chopped

⅓ cup (80 ml) fresh lemon juice

2 cups (480 ml) water (if blending), divided

THE METHOD

If you have a juicer, place the celery, lettuce, apples, parsley and cucumbers in the juicer and juice them according to the juicer's instructions. Pour the juice in a glass, add the lemon juice and serve the green juice.

If you don't have a juicer, combine half of celery, half of the lettuce, half of the apples, half of the parsley, half of the cucumber and 1 cup (240 ml) of the water in a high-powered blender. Blend the ingredients on high speed until everything is well combined. Pour the juice through a nut-milk straining bag over a large bowl, and strain out the juice by squeezing the contents in the bag with your hands. Repeat this process with the remaining celery, lettuce, apples, parsley, cucumber and 1 cup (240 ml) of water. Pour the liquid from the bowl in a glass, add the lemon juice and serve the green juice.

Make sure to drink this juice within 36 hours, as the longer you wait the more nutrients it loses.

BAI'S TIP: I give the leftover pulp to my pup—she loves it as an addition to her food! Such an easy way to boost your pup's nutrition.

If you want to switch up your juice, coarsely chop ½ medium pineapple and use that instead of the apples. You can also use cilantro instead of parsley and kale instead of romaine!

Yields 2 (32-oz [946-ml]) servings

GOLDEN HOUR JUICE

You're bound to feel glowing and golden after drinking this juice! This is a recipe packed with ingredients to make your skin glow and to strengthen your immune system. I am always looking for ways to pack nutrients into my day, and this is the (literally golden) ticket. Try drinking a full glass of water and then a 16-ounce (473-ml) cold-pressed juice first thing in the morning before your coffee, and you'll notice more energy, fewer blood sugar crashes, clearer skin and deeper sleep that night. You can also enjoy this as a mocktail that's perfect for a hot day: Use a ratio of 1 part Golden Hour Juice and 1 part bubbly water.

THE GOODS

½ medium pineapple, coarsely chopped

2 medium golden beets, peeled and coarsely chopped

3 tbsp (30 g) coarsely chopped fresh turmeric

3 tbsp (30 g) coarsely chopped fresh ginger

5 large carrots, finely chopped

4 large oranges, peeled

2 tbsp (30 ml) fresh lemon juice

1 cup (240 ml) water (if blending)

THE METHOD

In your juicer, combine the pineapple, beets, turmeric, ginger, carrots and oranges. Juice them according to the juicer's instructions. Transfer the juice to a glass, add the lemon juice and serve the golden juice.

If you don't have a juicer, combine the pineapple, beets, turmeric, ginger, carrots, oranges, lemon juice and water in a high-powered blender. Blend the ingredients until everything is smooth and combined. Pour the mixture through a nut-milk straining bag over a large bowl, then strain out the juice by squeezing the contents in the bag with your hands. You might want to wear gloves to avoid staining your hands with turmeric.

I love pouring this juice in a wine glass with some ice to complete the golden hour vibe!

BAI'S TIP: *I love to meal-prep this juice on Monday, so that I have enough to last for a few days. It's a great energy booster and will last for about 48 hours in your fridge. Avoid giving this pulp to your pup, as the ginger and pineapple are too much for canine systems.*

Yields 2 (20-oz [591-ml]) servings

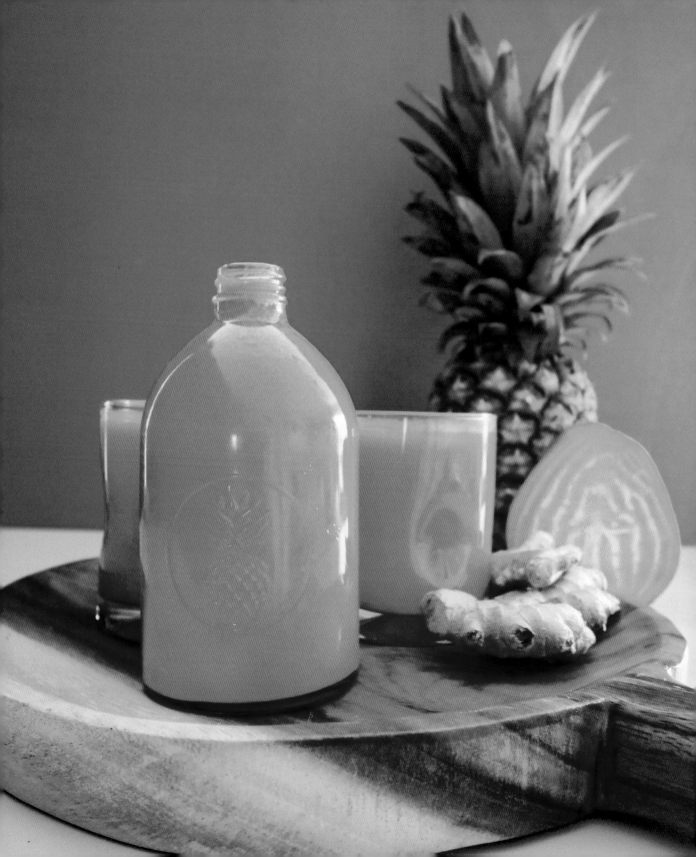

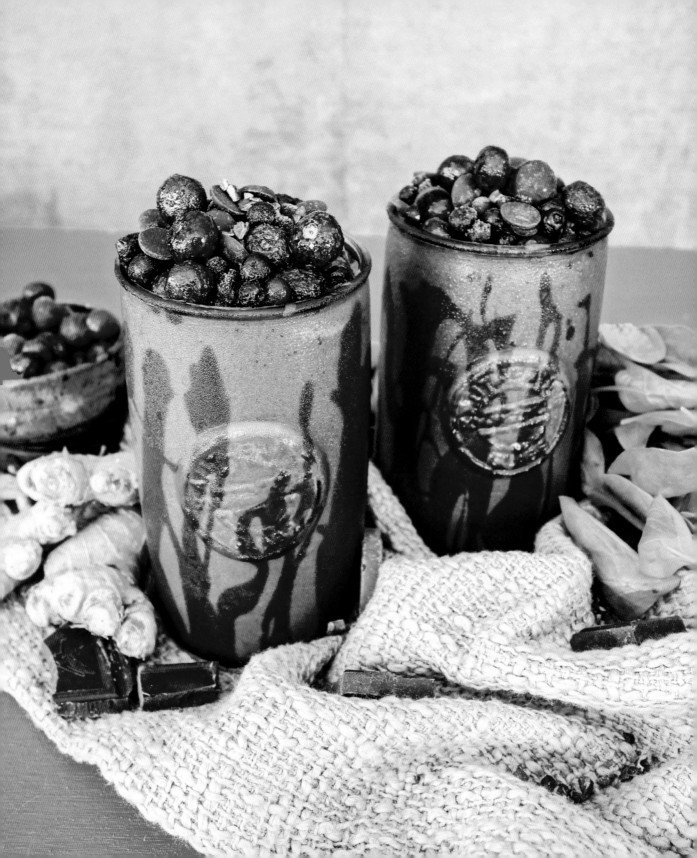

MIDNIGHT DREAM SMOOTHIE

Are you ready for the most delectable smoothie you've ever had? The mix of cacao, ginger and blueberries will give your morning a glorious start that will leave you happy, energized and ready for whatever your day brings. This immune-boosting powerhouse is the perfect thing to drink when you're on a coffee break, and it will help you manage anxiety and feel more open when you're experiencing stress. Not only that, but you'll get a high dose of antioxidants, healthy fats, protein, vitamin A, iron and magnesium, just to name a few. I had a smoothie just like this almost every day when I was traveling in Bali. My skin was glowing, and I was energized and calm. Although I could attribute that to Bali's magic, I will say that I took the idea of this smoothie home with me and it's now my secret weapon. The Midnight Dream is the just medicine you'll need on sleepy weekday mornings.

THE GOODS

2 packed cups (200 g) baby spinach

1 medium ripe fresh or frozen banana

½ cup (56 g) cacao powder

1 tbsp (6 g) peeled and thinly sliced ginger

½ cup (120 g) almond butter

3 cups (400 g) frozen blueberries

1 cup (240 ml) Cashew-Hemp Milk (page 162) or plant milk of choice

THE METHOD

In a high-powered blender, combine the spinach, banana, cacao, ginger, almond butter, blueberries and milk. Blend the ingredients on high speed until they are smooth. Take the smoothie to work with you or eat it slowly with a spoon!

BAI'S TIP: To make this smoothie a dream for your pleasure center, pour it in a bowl and top it with melted vegan chocolate, more frozen blueberries and almond butter. Yum!

Makes 2 (16-oz [473-ml]) servings

TROPICAL GREEN SMOOTHIE

My smoothies have come a long way since my early days of making them, but this one stays tried and true. This is the perfect entry-level green smoothie and can convince almost anyone to get down with some veggies. The tropical fruit helps boost your immunity while adding a delicious and natural sweetness to the smoothie. The hemp seeds are my favorite clean source of plant-based protein and omega-3. Coconut water is hydrating, is filled with potassium and also sweetens the deal. A quick tip: Check the ingredients when you're buying coconut water—look for varieties with no added sugars! Any way you flip the coin on this smoothie, you'll be so happy you made it for breakfast. Actually, this recipe works for almost any time you're feeling hungry and needing a quick nutrient boost. Keep these ingredients on hand, so that day or night you can blend your way to smoothie bliss.

THE GOODS

1 small cucumber, thickly sliced

2 small ribs celery, finely chopped

2 packed cups (200 g) baby spinach

1 cup (240 ml) coconut water

¼ cup (30 g) hemp seeds (see Bai's Tip)

1 cup (130 g) thickly sliced fresh or frozen pineapple

2 cups (280 g) frozen mango

THE METHOD

In a high-powered blender, combine the cucumber, celery, spinach, coconut water and hemp seeds. Blend the ingredients on high speed for about 1 minute. Blending the greens first makes for a velvety smoothie! Add the pineapple and mango. Blend the smoothie for 1 minute, pour it into two large glasses and serve it.

BAI'S TIP: I use hemp seeds as the protein here, but feel free to add your favorite dairy-free plain or vanilla protein powder, or add chia seeds and flax seeds for added protein.

Makes 2 (20-oz [591-ml]) servings

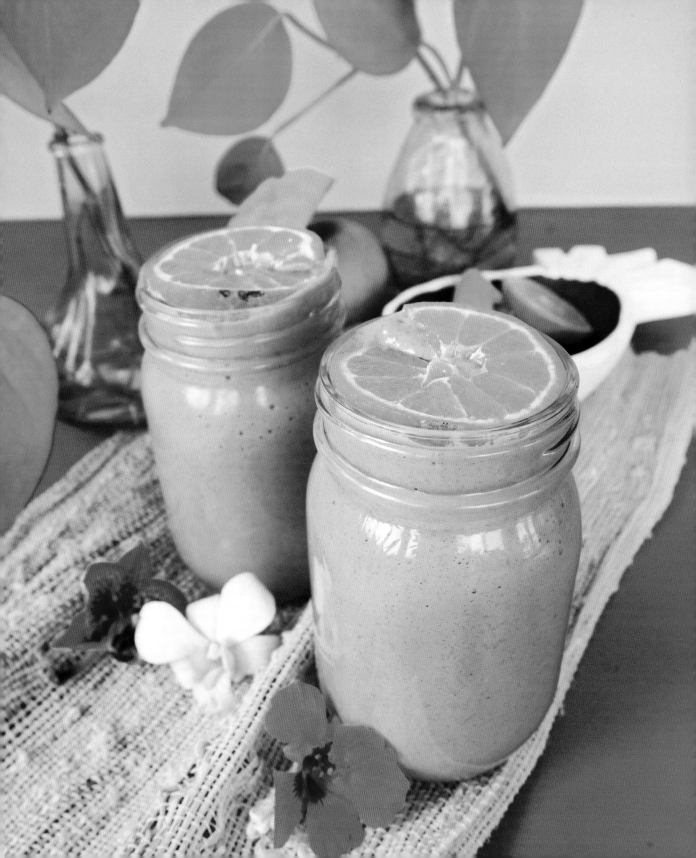

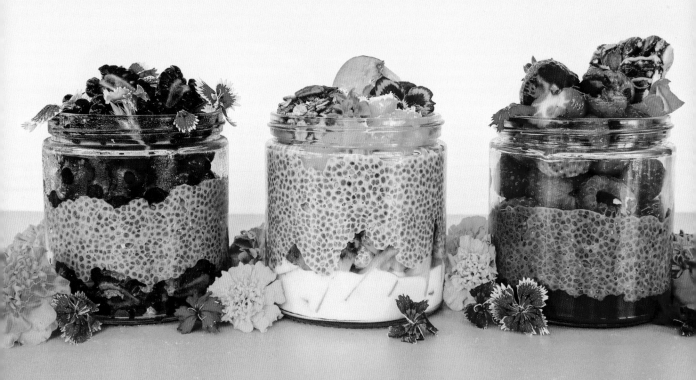

CHIA PUDDING THREE WAYS

Meal-prepping a breakfast that's delicious and gorgeous can get you hyped for your morning in a whole new way. These chia puddings are so simple to put together, and they hit the spot after you've been to the gym or while you're on your way to a meeting. This chia pudding is stocked with plant protein, boasting 5 grams in each little jar. It's clean food to get you pumped for your day, and it's ready for you in your fridge as a snack when you need it the most. Each of the following ingredient lists is meant to yield 1 (16-ounce [473-ml]) jar of pudding, so you can easily make as many servings as you need to set up your week.

THE GOODS

MATCHA CHIA PUDDING
¼ cup (40 g) chia seeds
½ tsp matcha powder
1 cup (240 ml) oat milk
1 to 2 tsp (5 to 10 ml) maple syrup
½ cup (67 g) fresh blueberries
¼ cup (33 g) fresh blackberries

MANGO-COCO CHIA PUDDING
¼ cup (40 g) chia seeds
1 cup (240 ml) coconut milk
¼ tsp pure vanilla extract
1 to 2 tsp (5 to 10 ml) maple syrup
¼ cup (41 g) coarsely chopped fresh or frozen mango
¼ cup (41 g) coarsely chopped fresh or frozen peaches
1 tsp unsweetened shredded coconut
¼ cup (30 g) granola of choice

CHOCOLATE COVERED–STRAWBERRY CHIA PUDDING
¼ cup (40 g) chia seeds
1 tsp cacao powder
1 cup (240 ml) oat milk
1 to 2 tsp (5 to 10 ml) maple syrup
½ cup (80 g) thickly sliced fresh strawberries
¼ cup (33 g) fresh raspberries
¼ cup (60 ml) melted dark chocolate
1 Pecan-Cacao Date Bar (page 144)

THE METHOD

Matcha Chia Pudding

Pour the chia seeds in the bottom of a 16-ounce (473-ml) jar. Add the matcha and mix the two well until the matcha coats all the chia seeds. Add the oat milk and maple syrup and mix the ingredients well with a fork to make the pudding smooth. You can add the blueberries and blackberries now, or wait until it has set and then place on top. Cover the jar with its lid and transfer it to the fridge. The pudding will be set in about 30 minutes. You may want to mix halfway through to avoid any clumps. Store the pudding, covered, in the fridge.

Mango-Coco Chia Pudding

Pour the chia seeds in the bottom of a 16-ounce (473-ml) jar. Add the coconut milk, vanilla and maple syrup and mix the ingredients well with a fork to make the pudding smooth. You can add the mango and peaches now, or wait until it has set and then place on top. Cover the jar with its lid and transfer it to the fridge. The pudding will be set in about 30 minutes. You may want to mix halfway through to avoid any clumps. Once your chia pudding has set, top it with the shredded coconut and granola. Store the pudding, covered, in the fridge.

Chocolate Covered–Strawberry Chia Pudding

Pour the chia seeds in the bottom of a 16-ounce (473-ml) jar with a lid. Add the cacao and mix well until the cacao coats all the chia seeds. Add the oat milk and maple syrup and mix the ingredients well with a fork to make the pudding smooth. You can add the strawberries and raspberries now, or wait until it has set and then place on top. Cover the jar with its lid and transfer it to the fridge. The pudding will be set in about 30 minutes. You may want to mix halfway through to avoid any clumps. Once the pudding is set, drizzle it with the dark chocolate. Or grab a clean 16-ounce (473-ml) jar and pour the chocolate in the bottom, then add the chia pudding, strawberries and raspberries. Dunk the date bar into the top of the pudding. Store the pudding, covered, in the fridge.

Makes 1 (16-oz [473-ml]) jar of each pudding

CARAMEL APPLE OATMEAL

Caramel apples are the ultimate food at the fair or the boardwalk. In the '90s, I grew up with those snack packs of caramel sauce for apple slices and damn, they were so good. The love for caramel will never perish—it's all about reinventing the way we make it. Traditional caramel sauce has butter, heavy whipping cream and white sugar, which is not the vibe we want when we're looking at food from a healing perspective. Luckily, we can re-create a caramel sauce using four simple ingredients from the plant world to make a refined sugar–free, dairy-free version that's an amazing option for kids and adults alike. I add this caramel sauce to some oats and cooked apples, as I figure life is too short not to have caramel first thing in the morning. It's the perfect time of day to create new food memories for you and your kids.

THE GOODS

OATMEAL
1 cup (240 ml) water

1 cup (240 ml) Cashew-Hemp Milk (page 162) or plant milk of choice

½ tsp pure vanilla extract

¼ tsp salt

1 cup (90 g) rolled oats

1 large apple (any variety works well), finely chopped

2 tsp (6 g) coconut sugar

¼ tsp ground cinnamon

CARAMEL SAUCE
½ cup (120 g) almond butter

¼ tsp ground cinnamon

2 tbsp (30 ml) pure date or maple syrup

½ cup (120 ml) Cashew-Hemp Milk (page 162) or plant milk of choice

GARNISHES
1 large apple, thinly sliced

¼ cup (25 g) pecans

Unsweetened coconut flakes

THE METHOD

First, make the oatmeal. In medium saucepan over medium-low heat, combine the water, milk, vanilla and salt. Bring the mixture to a light boil. Once the mixture is boiling, add the oats, apple, sugar and cinnamon. Reduce the heat to low and cook the oatmeal for 10 minutes, stirring it occasionally, until the liquid is absorbed and the oats are tender.

While your oats are cooking, make the caramel sauce. In another small saucepan over medium heat, combine the almond butter, cinnamon and date syrup. Stir the ingredients with a rubber spatula for 30 seconds to mix them well. Slowly pour in the milk and cook the sauce for 1 minute, stirring it constantly, until it is smooth.

Remove both the oats and the caramel sauce from the heat. Evenly distribute the oatmeal and cooked apple between two small serving bowls. Drizzle the caramel sauce over the oatmeal, and then garnish each serving with the apple, pecans and coconut flakes. Serve the oatmeal immediately.

BAI'S TIP: Meal-prep this recipe for your busy workdays or a road trip. Cook the caramel sauce as directed. Instead of cooking the oats, pour 1 cup (90 g) of oats into two small Mason jars. Add the cinnamon, coconut sugar and vanilla to each jar and mix the ingredients well. Cover the oats with the milk, then add the apples and a drizzle of the caramel. Let the oatmeal sit in the fridge for 2 hours or overnight, and you've got yourself a five-star breakfast on the road!

Makes 2 servings

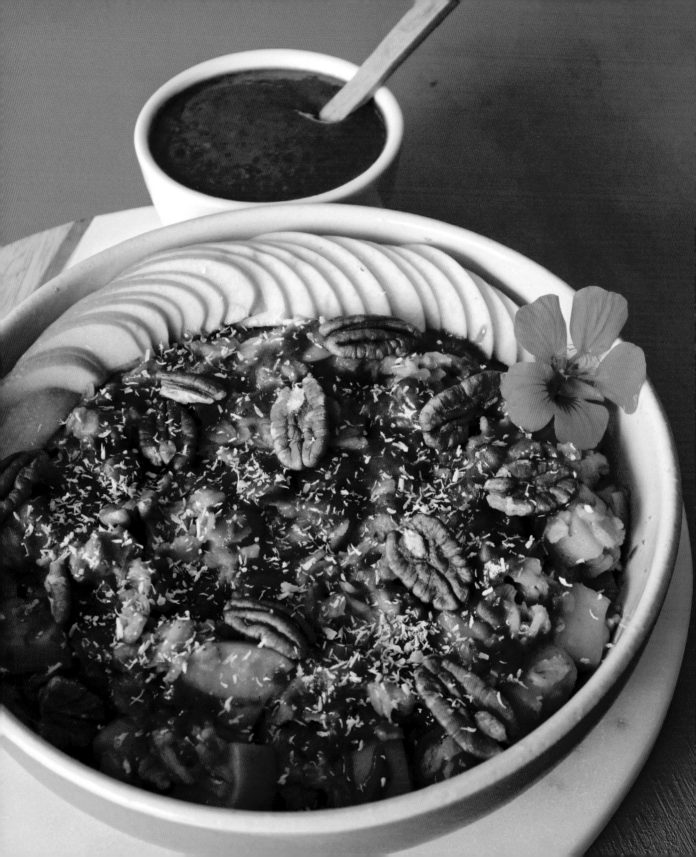

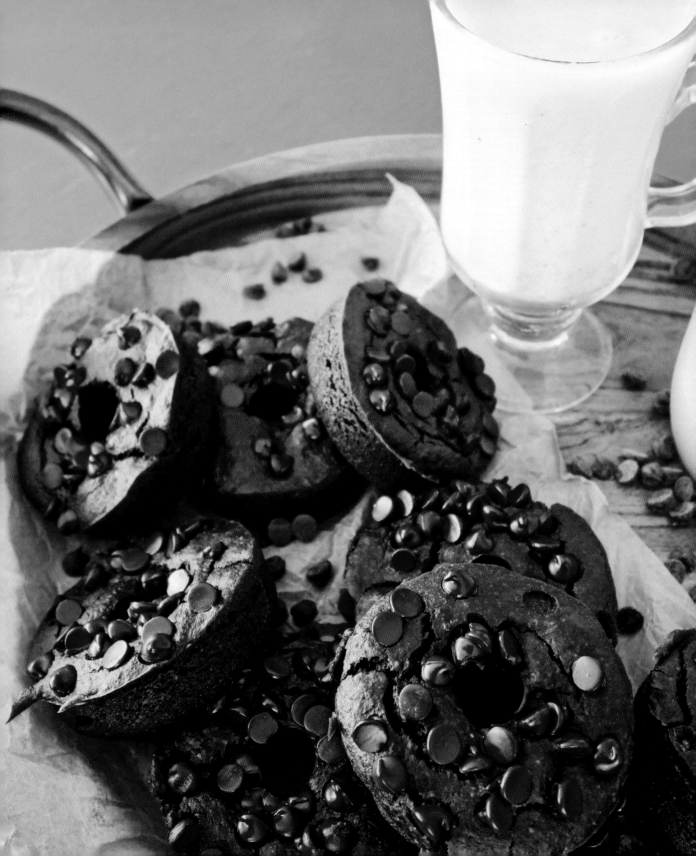

BLENDER DARK CHOCOLATE DONUTS

Holy chocolate deliciousness! I had to flip a coin on whether this recipe should appear in this chapter or in the sweets chapter, as these are so good they could easily pass as dessert. For the sake of experiencing culinary pleasure throughout the day, breakfast takes the cake for these donuts. I have been making these for years on retreats and for clients, and they are the favorite every single time. I've even looked into what it would take to get these on grocery store shelves, they're that good. For now, you'll just have to make these yourself and get lost in how truly delicious a plant-based treat can be. These little gems are a hybrid of brownies, muffins, donuts and zucchini bread. It really doesn't get much better. All you do is blend, bake and dive in! Easy as that.

THE GOODS

2 tbsp (30 ml) melted coconut oil

2 tbsp (12 g) ground chia seeds

¼ cup (60 ml) water

1 cup (90 g) rolled oats

1 cup (100 g) shredded zucchini

½ cup (80 g) coconut sugar

½ cup (120 g) almond butter

2 medium ripe bananas, peeled

1 tsp baking soda

½ cup (56 g) cacao powder

¼ tsp salt

1 tsp pure vanilla extract

1 cup (170 g) dark chocolate chips, divided

THE METHOD

Preheat the oven to 350°F (177°C). Prepare two six-cavity silicone or metal donut pans or muffin pans by greasing the cavities with the oil.

In a small bowl, mix together the chia seeds and water to make a chia egg. Let the chia egg set for 5 minutes.

Grab a high-powered blender and place the oats in the blender. Blend the oats for 20 seconds, until you get a powder. Add the chia egg, zucchini, sugar, almond butter, bananas, baking soda, cacao, salt, vanilla and ½ cup (85 g) of the chocolate chips. Blend the ingredients for about 1 minute, until you get a smooth batter. Pour the batter in each donut cavity until it evenly hits the top of the cavity. Top the donuts with the remaining ½ cup (85 g) of chocolate chips.

Bake the donuts for 15 to 18 minutes. If you are making muffins, bake them for 18 minutes. You'll know they are done when you press on the top of a donut and it bounces back and doesn't sink in.

Immediately remove the donuts from the pans by flipping each pan upside down onto a plate or the countertop. Transfer the donuts to a wire rack to cool.

Makes 1 dozen donuts

BLUEBERRY CINNAMON ROLLS
WITH MAPLE CREAM CHEESE ICING

You're about to reach a new level of breakfast deliciousness with this recipe! It's a combination of two of my favorite classics: the blueberry muffin and the cinnamon roll. Cinnamon rolls are no doubt a labor of love and so incredibly worth it! These are transformed from your typical cinnamon roll by the blueberry sauce, the spelt flour, the coconut sugar and this amazing cream cheese icing—no powdered sugar needed. I added spelt to this recipe to show you how truly versatile this flour can be. This is a cinnamon roll that will still give you a sugar rush, but save you from the bloat and the puffiness that are the results of a typical roll made with refined white flour and refined white sugar. This is the perfect recipe for holidays, celebrations or whenever you just need a good ol' cinnamon roll with a twist. Fill your house with the blissful aroma of cinnamon and master your morning in a whole new way!

THE GOODS

DOUGH

1 tbsp (9 g) active dry yeast

4 tbsp (40 g) coconut sugar, divided

1 cup (240 ml) Cashew-Hemp Milk (page 162) or unsweetened plant milk, warmed to about 105°F (41°C)

¼ cup (60 ml) melted Not Your Mama's Salted Butter (page 158) or store-bought vegan butter

2¼ cups (360 g) spelt flour, plus more as needed

BLUEBERRY SAUCE

1½ cups (200 g) frozen blueberries

¼ cup (60 ml) pure maple syrup

¼ cup (60 ml) fresh orange juice

1 tbsp (15 ml) fresh lemon juice

2 tbsp (18 g) tapioca flour

THE METHOD

Make the dough first. In a large bowl, combine the yeast, 1 tablespoon (10 g) of the sugar and the milk. Let this mixture sit for 10 minutes to allow the yeast to bloom and get foamy. Add the butter and the remaining 3 tablespoons (30 g) of sugar. Mix the ingredients well, and then start to incorporate the flour 1 cup (160 g) at a time with a wooden spoon. A dough will form. Knead it five or six times, until the flour is absorbed and you have a perfect-looking dough ball. Cover the dough with a warm, slightly damp dish towel and let it rise for 40 minutes, until it has almost doubled in size.

While your dough is rising, make your blueberry sauce. In a medium saucepan over medium heat, combine the blueberries, maple syrup, orange juice and lemon juice. Cook the mixture for about 10 minutes, mixing the ingredients with a whisk and smashing the blueberries with the whisk while they cook. At the last 2 minutes of cooking, whisk in the tapioca flour. Remove the saucepan from the heat and set it aside to cool.

Preheat your oven to 375°F (191°C). Lightly dust a work surface with spelt flour.

Remove the dough from the bowl and place it on the prepared work surface. Sprinkle a small amount of spelt flour on the top of the dough ball. Roll the dough out into a rectangle that is ½ inch (1.3 cm) thick.

(continued)

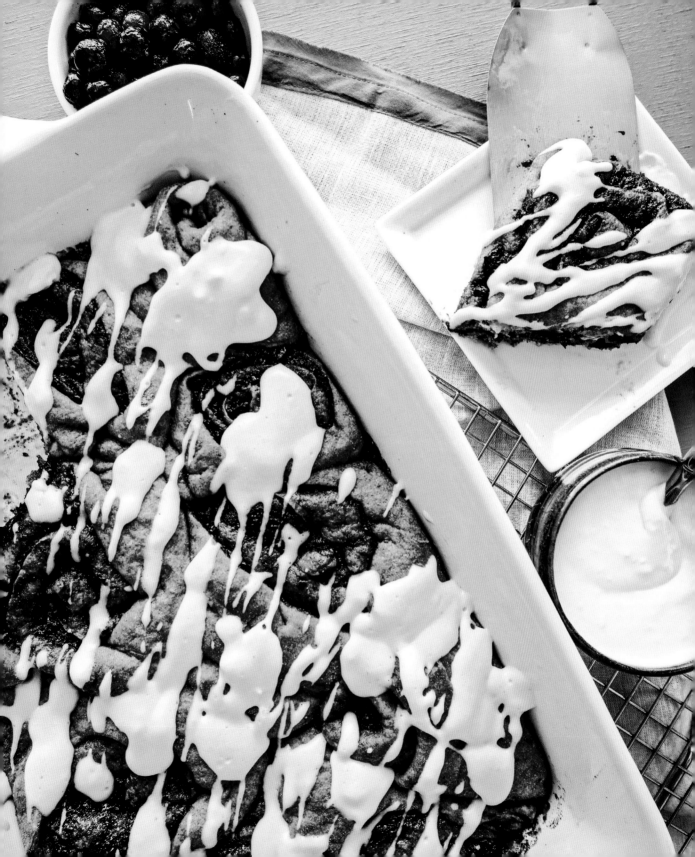

CINNAMON FILLING

¼ cup (60 ml) melted Not Your Mama's Salted Butter (page 158) or store-bought vegan butter, divided

2 tbsp (18 g) ground cinnamon

1 cup (160 g) coconut sugar

BUTTER AND MILK WASH

3 tbsp (45 ml) melted Not Your Mama's Salted Butter (page 158) or store-bought vegan butter

3 tbsp (45 ml) room-temperature plant milk

MAPLE CREAM CHEESE ICING

1 (8-oz [227-g]) package vegan cream cheese

¼ cup (60 ml) pure maple syrup

3 tbsp (45 ml) plant milk

1 tsp pure vanilla extract

Now it's time to create the cinnamon filling. Brush 3 tablespoons (45 ml) of the butter across the entire top of the dough. Then sprinkle the cinnamon and sugar all over the top of the buttered dough. Grab the blueberry sauce and spoon dollops of the sauce evenly around the cinnamon filling. Use your spoon to spread the blueberry sauce to create an even layer. Using the remaining 1 tablespoon (15 ml) of butter, grease a 9 x 13-inch (23 x 33–cm) baking dish. Set the baking dish within arm's reach of the dough.

Start to roll the dough on the long side. Roll evenly along the entire dough rectangle until you've rolled it completely. Using a sharp knife or a piece of unflavored dental floss, cut about 10 (2-inch [5-cm]-thick) rolls. Arrange the rolls in the prepared baking dish so that their cut sides are facing upward. Cover the rolls with the damp dish towel and let them rise for 20 minutes.

While the rolls are rising, make the butter and milk wash. In a small bowl, whisk together the butter and the milk. After the rolls have risen, brush the butter and milk wash over them to coat the tops.

Bake the cinnamon rolls for 15 to 20 minutes, or until the tops are just turning golden brown in some spots.

While the rolls are baking, make your maple cream cheese icing. You can do this in the bowl of a stand mixer fitted with the whisk attachment, or you can do it the old-fashioned way in a medium bowl with a handheld whisk. In the bowl, combine the cream cheese, maple syrup, milk and vanilla. Whisk until the ingredients are well combined.

Cover the rolls with all that gorgeous icing and serve them while they are warm.

Makes 10 cinnamon rolls

BREAKFAST TACOS WITH RANCHERO SAUCE

Tacos for every meal? Hell, yeah. Breakfast tacos are a whole vibe: They're super easy to put together, they're so flavorful, they're perfect for brunch and they're a great pairing with a Bloody Maria, a Bloody Mary with tequila. This ranchero sauce is excellent on enchiladas or as a salsa with chips, so make sure to bookmark this recipe for other occasions besides breakfast. To make this recipe huevos rancheros–style, you can assemble the tortillas close together on a plate, scoop some of the tofu scramble mixture on the tortillas, smother everything with hot ranchero sauce and drizzle some Cashew Cream (page 173) on top. You can make everything as part of your meal prep, since leftover tofu scrambles don't get weird like leftover eggs do! This is just one recipe with so many different ways to enjoy it.

THE GOODS

TACOS

1 tsp olive oil

1 medium sweet potato, thinly sliced

½ medium yellow onion, thinly sliced

1 tsp salt

Splash plus ¼ cup (60 ml) Immune-Boosting Veggie Broth (page 170), divided

1 cup (80 g) thinly sliced cremini mushrooms

½ tsp granulated garlic

¼ tsp black pepper

1 (14-oz [397-g]) block firm tofu, drained

1 tsp ground turmeric

½ tsp black salt

10 corn tortillas

Thinly sliced radishes, for garnish

Finely chopped fresh cilantro, for garnish

Avocado slices, for garnish

THE METHOD

First, begin preparing the tacos. Heat the oil in a large sauté pan over medium-high heat. Throw in the sweet potato, onion and salt. Cook the vegetables for 7 to 10 minutes, stirring them often, until the sweet potato is semisoft. Use a splash of broth if the mixture starts to stick or burn at any point. Add the mushrooms, granulated garlic and black pepper and cook the mixture for 2 minutes, until the mushrooms shrink in size. Mix in the remaining ¼ cup (60 ml) of broth to deglaze the pan. Next, use your hands to crumble the tofu into small pieces over the pan. Sprinkle the turmeric and black salt over the tofu and mix everything together well. Reduce the heat to low and cook the tofu scramble for 3 to 5 minutes, stirring it occasionally. Remove the pan from the heat and cover it to keep the scramble warm.

(continued)

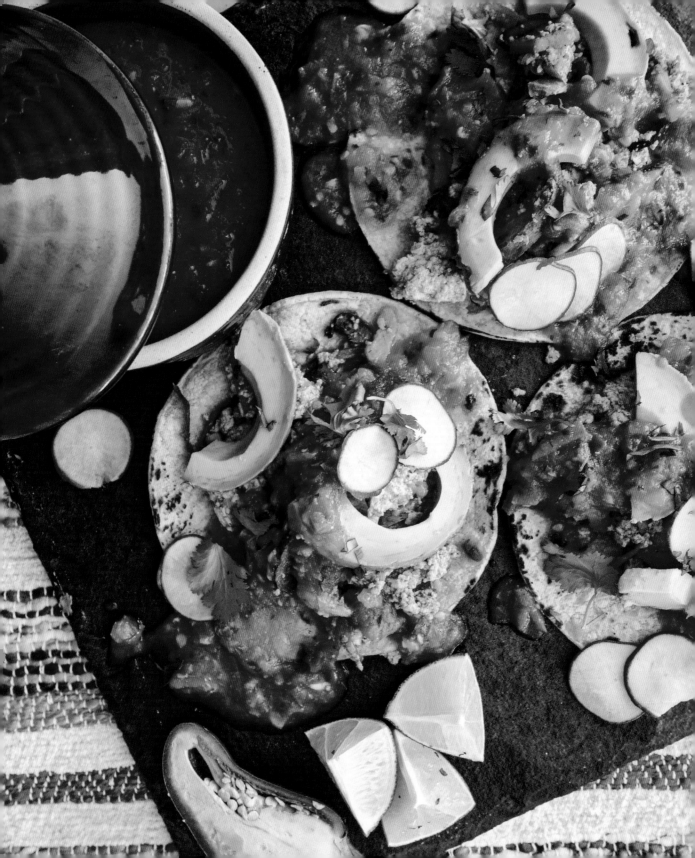

RANCHERO SAUCE

1 tsp olive oil

½ medium yellow onion, diced

¾ tsp salt, divided

2 cloves garlic, minced

1 (4-oz [113-g]) can mild green chilies, undrained

½ small jalapeño pepper, thinly sliced

2 large tomatoes, diced

½ tsp ground cumin

½ tsp paprika

1 tsp fresh lime juice

¼ packed cup (30 g) fresh cilantro, minced

While you're cooking your scramble, make the ranchero sauce. Grab a small saucepan and heat oil over medium-high heat. Add the onion and ¼ teaspoon of the salt and cook the mixture for 2 to 3 minutes. Toss in the garlic, remaining ½ teaspoon of salt and green chilies with their juice. Cook the mixture for 1 minute, and then stir in the jalapeño, tomatoes, cumin and paprika. Cooking in layers like this will add a lot of depth to your sauce versus cooking it all at once. Stir the sauce, cover the saucepan, reduce the heat to medium and cook the sauce for 7 to 10 minutes. If you prefer a chunky sauce, simmer it for another 10 minutes. If you prefer a smooth sauce, transfer the sauce to a blender and blend or pulse until the sauce reaches your desired consistency. Next, add the lime juice and cilantro. If you have blended your sauce, return it to the saucepan. Cover the saucepan and set it aside to keep the sauce warm.

To put it all together, heat your tortillas by cooking them over the open flame of your stove for 30 seconds on each side, until they are brown on the edges. If you have an electric stove, heat a dry large cast-iron skillet over medium-high heat. Heat the tortillas for 30 seconds on each side. Transfer them to a tortilla warmer to steam. Grab a few plates and place 2 to 3 tortillas on each plate. Top the tortillas with the tofu scramble, ranchero sauce, radishes, cilantro and avocado. Serve the breakfast tacos immediately with a Bloody Maria!

Makes 10 tacos

FLUFFY FLOURLESS ACAI PANCAKES

These pancakes are fuss-free, are super easy to make and stay with you all morning. The biggest complaint I hear about pancakes is that they don't keep you full long enough, and I couldn't agree more! Oats and bananas are filled with fiber and are the main ingredients in this recipe, which will keep you satisfied and full for hours. The added acai is a superfood boost to these already nutritious pancakes. Make the batter ahead of time over the weekend and store it in a blender bottle for easy pouring when you are in a hurry during the week! Just heat the pan, shake up the batter, pour it out and—voilà!—you've got fluffy pancakes on Monday morning.

THE GOODS

PANCAKES

2 medium ripe bananas, peeled

2 cups (180 g) rolled oats

½ cup (120 ml) Cashew-Hemp Milk (page 162) or plant milk of choice

1 tbsp (12 g) baking powder

1½ tbsp (23 ml) apple cider vinegar

¾ cup (60 g) acai concentrate (see Bai's Tip)

3 tbsp (45 ml) pure maple syrup

1 tbsp (15 ml) melted coconut oil

OPTIONAL TOPPINGS

Not Your Mama's Salted Butter (page 158) or store-bought vegan butter

Pure maple syrup

Berries

Vegan whipped cream

THE METHOD

In a high-powered blender or food processor, combine the bananas, oats, milk, baking powder, vinegar, acai concentrate and maple syrup. Blend the ingredients until they are smooth. The batter will be a thick mixture, so be patient. Use your blender's accelerator stick or use a spatula to scrape down the sides of the food processor's bowl.

In a large skillet, heat the oil over low heat. Once the oil and pan are hot, add ¼ cup (60 ml) of the batter to the skillet and spread the batter around to make a pancake. Repeat this process until you have a few pancakes in the skillet with enough room to easily flip each one. Cook the pancakes for about 1 minute on each side—you'll know the first side is done when the pancake starts to bubble on the top and easily comes away from the skillet. Flip the pancakes with a spatula. Repeat this process until you use up all the pancake batter.

Serve a few pancakes on each individual plate, or make a huge stack to share with a friend! Top the pancakes with any or all of the optional toppings: butter, maple syrup, berries and whipped cream. Serve the pancakes immediately.

BAI'S TIP: You can find frozen acai packets in the freezer section by the frozen fruit! If you can't find acai or want to try something else, just use ¾ cup (180 g) of your favorite fruit or berries or ¾ cup (180 ml) of melted chocolate.

Makes 6 to 7 pancakes

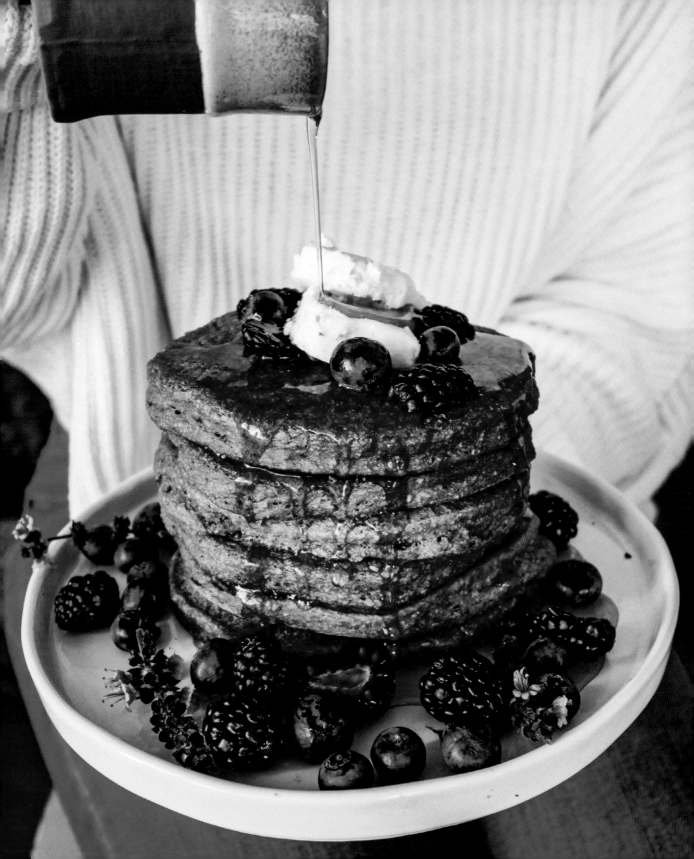

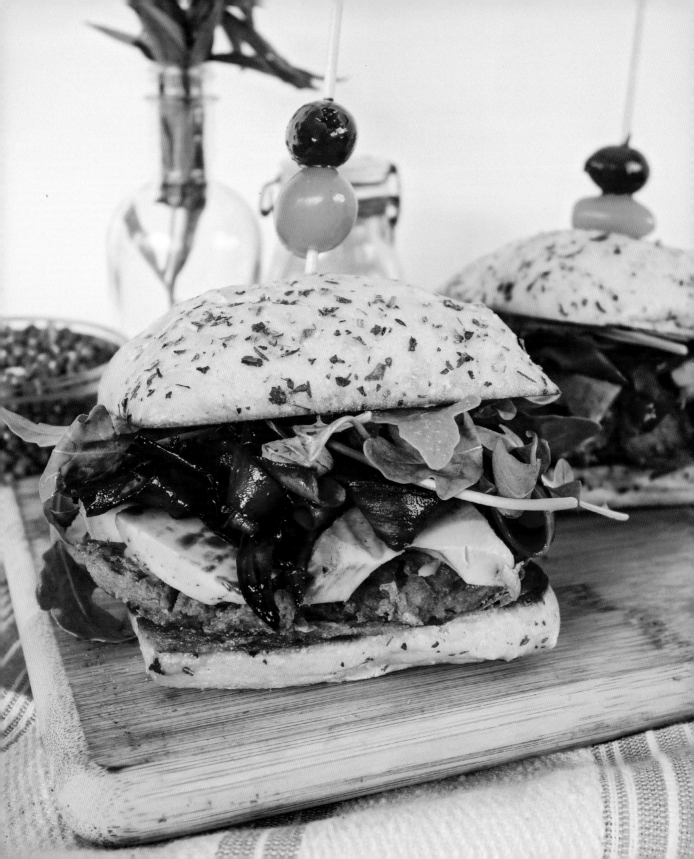

THE ULTIMATE BREAKFAST SANDO

Drool-worthy just got a whole new meaning with this one. This is everything you could want in a breakfast sandwich and then some. The egg is super clean protein from moong dal or sprouted mung beans (look for them at the grocery store where you would find lentils), and—unlike eggs, which are packed with cholesterol—these little guys actually can help lower your cholesterol and improve your circulation. The bacon marinates really quickly and is the perfect addition to this sandwich, without any of the scary health risks you take when you eat animal-based bacon. Load up ciabatta buns with the heart-healthy eggs, bacon, avocado, melty cheese and arugula—you get what you want and what you need, all wrapped up into one glorious breakfast sammie.

THE GOODS

EGG

1 cup (115 g) moong dal or sprouted mung beans

Boiling water, as needed

1 cup (240 ml) unsweetened plant milk

¼ cup (30 g) quinoa flour

½ tsp table or Himalayan pink salt

½ tsp black salt

½ tsp garlic powder

½ tsp onion powder

½ tsp ground turmeric

1 tsp olive oil

BACON

2 large carrots, peeled into strips

1 tbsp (15 ml) agave nectar

2 tbsp (30 ml) coconut aminos

2 tbsp (30 ml) liquid smoke

1 tbsp (15 ml) liquid aminos

SANDOS

3 ciabatta buns

Not Your Mama's Salted Butter (page 158) or store-bought vegan butter, as needed

3 tsp (15 g) Dijon mustard

½ cup (50 g) shredded vegan Cheddar cheese

1½ cups (45 g) arugula

1 medium avocado, thickly sliced

THE METHOD

First, begin preparing the egg by soaking the moong dal beans. Place the beans in a heatproof medium bowl and pour the boiling water over them. Let the moong dal soak for 15 to 20 minutes.

While the moong dal beans soak, begin preparing the bacon. Place the carrot strips in a medium bowl. In a small Mason jar, mix together the agave, coconut aminos, liquid smoke and liquid aminos. Pour the marinade over the carrot strips and let them marinate while you wait for your moong dal beans to soak.

Once your moong dal beans have soaked, drain them and rinse them with fresh water. Place the beans in a blender and add the milk, flour, table salt, black salt, garlic powder, onion powder and turmeric. Blend the ingredients until the batter is super smooth. Heat a large nonstick sauté pan over medium-high heat and add the oil. Once the oil is hot, pour your egg mixture evenly over the bottom of the pan. Cook the egg for about 1 minute, and then slowly release it from the bottom of the pan with a rubber spatula. Treat the egg as scrambled eggs and keep folding and releasing the egg from the bottom of the pan for 5 to 7 minutes, until the egg is fully cooked. Cover the pan to keep the egg warm.

Heat a medium skillet over medium-high heat. Add the marinated carrots and cook them for about 5 minutes, until they're crispy on the outside. Remove the bacon from the skillet and keep the skillet over the heat.

To make the sandos, cut your ciabatta buns in half and spread the inside of each half with about 1 teaspoon of the butter. Toast the buns in the skillet for about 20 seconds, until the inside of each is golden brown.

Make your sandwiches by spreading 1 teaspoon of the mustard on the bottom half of each bun. Then add one-third of the egg mixture to each bun. Next, top the egg with the Cheddar cheese, arugula, avocado, bacon and the top half of the bun.

Makes 3 sandwiches

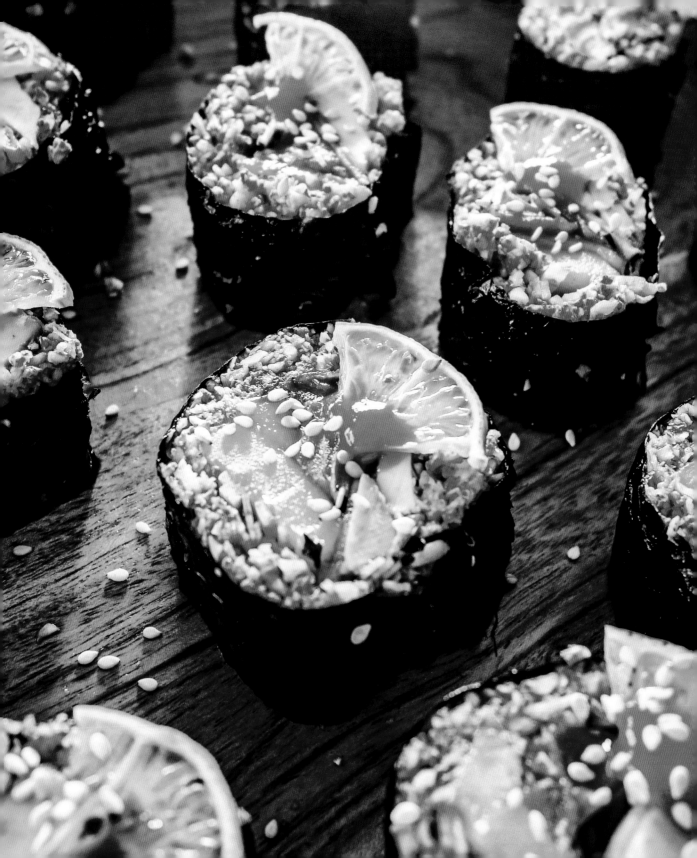

MIDDAY *Munchies*

Life is too short for boring salads and the same turkey sandwich you've been eating for 25 years. Life is about truly enjoying yourself, even if it's just lunch on a Tuesday. It's the simple and seemingly mundane moments when we feel most alive that give our lives so much meaning. Seems like a tall order for lunch, but I am on a mission to change the cultural assumption that nothing really matters besides working, making money and trying to "fit it all in" between the hours of 9:00 a.m. and 5:00 p.m. Monday through Friday.

Somewhere amid the clamor of consumer culture, the drive-through and being able to work right from our phone, we lost the idea of sitting down every day to actually enjoy all three meals. I envy cultures in Europe who close up shop for two hours to eat, nap and, you know, just be human. We've lost the humanity in our workdays, and a perfect symbol of that is how and what we eat for lunch.

Don't get me wrong, there are some people and tech companies who have it figured out. The majority of us, though, could use a little assistance in making ourselves a priority during this crucial time in our day. All of your current realities aside, what would your life look like if you had your ideal lunch hour? How would it change your life? Your relationships? Your relationship to stress? We can accomplish a lot by changing a little about how we do things every day.

Something simple you can do over the weekend is decide how you want to fully enjoy your next lunch hour. Maybe you'd like to eat under a tree, on the beach or at a new restaurant you've been dying to try. Maybe the reality is that you are just too damn busy and what would really help is a delicious and satisfying meal that gives you the energy you need. That's what this chapter is designed to do—help you be your absolute best self. These recipes are simple, flavorful and designed with you in mind. I love the Rustic Italian Chopped Salad (page 130) when I'm on the go. I also like to make a big pot of the Moroccan Lentil Soup (page 137) to last the whole week. Remember, you can do it all and take care of yourself too! Get down on these midday munchies and get what you need to slay the rest of your day.

CURRIED COCONUT LENTIL SALAD

My love affair with lentils is one of my favorite parts of being plant-based. In the past, I never gave lentils the love and attention they deserve. I would always order something else on the menu or go for other legumes instead. These days, it's a whole different story. Lentils are one of the most amazing things you can eat for your health. Per serving, lentils actually have more iron than ground beef with just as much protein, none of the saturated fat and a tiny fraction of carbon emissions. Not too bad for some little legumes! This salad is complete with roasted veggies, baby kale and a dressing that'll knock your socks off. Let this salad give you a chance to go outside of your daily norm for an Indian-inspired treat!

THE GOODS

SALAD

3 cups (720 ml) Immune-Boosting Veggie Broth (page 170)

1 cup (200 g) red lentils, rinsed

3 cups (300 g) cauliflower florets

8 medium broccolini tops

1 medium orange bell pepper, thinly sliced

2 tbsp (30 ml) olive oil

1 tsp salt

½ tsp black pepper

½ tsp ground turmeric

½ tsp ground ginger

½ tsp ground cinnamon

1 (5-oz [142-g]) package baby kale

2 tbsp (16 g) roasted salted pumpkin seeds

DRESSING

¼ cup (60 g) unsweetened coconut yogurt (see Bai's Tip on page 169)

2 tbsp (30 g) vegan red curry paste

2 tbsp (30 ml) pure maple syrup

2 tbsp (30 ml) fresh lemon juice

2 tbsp (30 ml) water

¼ tsp salt

¼ tsp black pepper

THE METHOD

To make the salad, preheat the oven to 375°F (191°C).

While the oven is preheating, combine the broth and lentils in a small saucepan over medium-high heat. Bring the lentils to a boil, cover the saucepan and reduce the heat to low. Simmer the lentils for 10 to 15 minutes, stirring them occasionally, until they are tender but not mushy.

While the lentils are cooking, place the cauliflower, broccolini and bell pepper on a large baking sheet. Add the oil, salt, black pepper, turmeric, ginger and cinnamon and toss everything together with your hands. Bake the vegetables for 12 to 15 minutes, until the broccolini is dark green and the cauliflower is turning golden brown.

Now you can make the dressing. In a small bowl or Mason jar, whisk together the yogurt, curry paste, maple syrup, lemon juice, water, salt and black pepper until the dressing is smooth.

Assemble your salad. Layer the baby kale, lentils, roasted veggies and pumpkin seeds on a large serving tray or in three or four individual bowls. Finish the salad by drizzling the dressing on top. Serve the salad immediately.

BAI'S TIP: Make this into a Mason jar salad by grabbing three 32-ounce (907-g) Mason jars. Pour the dressing in on the bottoms of the jars first. Then add the lentils directly to the dressing. Add the roasted veggies and top it off with your baby kale and pumpkin seeds! Put the lids on the jars, refrigerate the salads and enjoy them within 5 to 6 days.

Makes 3 to 4 servings

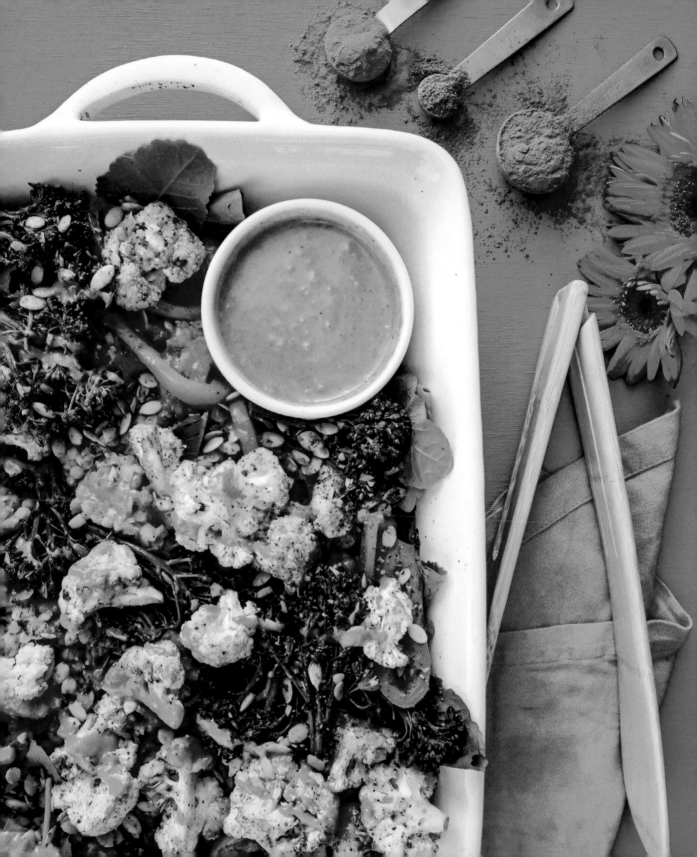

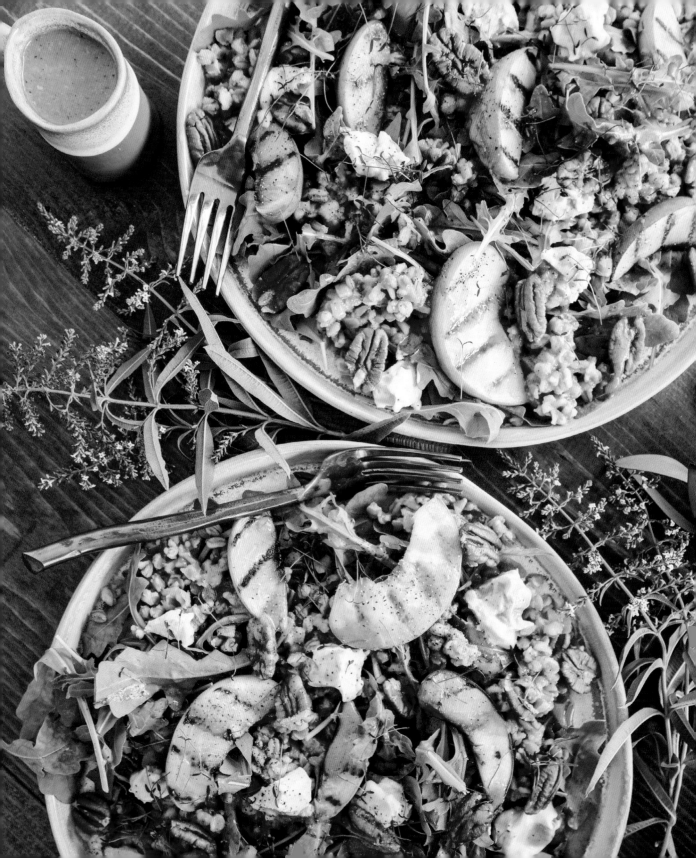

GRILLED STONE FRUIT FARRO SALAD

There's nothing quite like the taste of sweet summer: berries, peaches, nectarines and tan lines to match. The essence of summer is right here in this salad between the arugula, the raspberry vinaigrette and the grilled stone fruit. Living in San Diego has taught me that the endless summer is truly a mindset. Although eleven months of sun definitely helps, what I've learned is not to take life too seriously, to enjoy the little things and that surfing on your lunch break is wildly accepted and encouraged. If only all of us could take on a little more of this endless summer energy all year long. This recipe is deliciously seasonal, helping you savor and enjoy it that much more. This salad might not exactly be equal to surfing on your lunch break, but it's pretty damn close!

THE GOODS

FARRO
3 cups (720 ml) Immune-Boosting Veggie Broth (page 170)
½ tsp salt
1 cup (170 g) farro, rinsed

RASPBERRY VINAIGRETTE
¼ cup (33 g) raspberries
3 tbsp (45 ml) fresh lemon juice
1 tsp mustard powder
1 tbsp (15 ml) white wine vinegar
½ tsp salt
½ tsp black pepper
1 tbsp (15 ml) olive oil
1 tbsp (15 ml) agave nectar
2 tbsp (30 ml) water

SALAD
2 large stone fruits (such as peaches, apricots or nectarines), thickly sliced
1 (5-oz [142-g]) package arugula
½ cup (90 g) crumbled Herbed Creamy Feta (page 166) or store-bought vegan feta cheese

THE METHOD

First, prepare the farro. In a small saucepan over high heat, bring the broth to a boil. Add salt and farro. Cover the saucepan, reduce the heat to low and simmer the farro for 30 minutes, until it is al dente. If there is any liquid remaining in the saucepan, drain it.

While the farro is cooking, make the raspberry vinaigrette. In a blender, combine the raspberries, lemon juice, mustard powder, vinegar, salt, black pepper, oil, agave and water. Blend the ingredients until they are smooth. Set the vinaigrette aside.

To make the salad, preheat a grill to medium-high heat or heat a seasoned medium cast-iron grill pan over medium-high heat. Sear the sliced stone fruits for 2 minutes on each side, until golden-brown grill marks appear. If you are using a grill, make sure to arrange the slices of fruit in the opposite direction of the grates, so they don't fall through.

Now it's time to assemble the salad. Set out three or four serving plates. Divide the arugula among the plates. Top each serving of arugula with ¾ cup (150 g) of the farro, the Herbed Creamy Feta and the grilled stone fruit. Drizzle the raspberry vinaigrette over the top of each serving and serve the salad immediately.

BAI'S TIP: *Enjoy this recipe during the winter by swapping out the grilled stone fruits for grilled pears and the raspberries for pomegranate seeds.*

Makes 3 to 4 servings

THE VIBRANT ROLL

When California vibes meet Japanese umami flavors, you get something magical that looks a bit like this. Vegan sushi is the future not only because it's delicious, but also because if we're not careful, it's the only memory of the fish in the oceans we'll have left. The fishing industries are so detrimental to ocean life, and as consumers, it's our job to stay educated so that we can shop, cook and eat responsibly to protect ocean life and our environment. You'll need a sushi mat for this recipe, and if you're a newbie—patience is key. The more you do, the better you'll get! I've included cauliflower rice for a lighter, more nutrient-dense twist. This roll is vibrant, refreshing and sustainable.

THE GOODS

CAULIFLOWER RICE
1 large head purple cauliflower, cut into florets
1 tbsp (15 ml) plain rice vinegar
1 tbsp (15 ml) fresh lemon juice

TOMATO TUNA
3 medium hothouse tomatoes
1 tbsp (15 ml) toasted sesame oil
2 tbsp (30 ml) liquid aminos
2 tbsp (30 ml) coconut aminos
1 tbsp (15 ml) plain rice vinegar

ROLLS
½ medium cucumber, thinly sliced
½ medium avocado, thickly sliced
½ medium mango, peeled and thinly sliced
1 medium radish, thinly sliced
4 sheets nori

GARNISHES
Sliced pickled ginger
Liquid aminos or soy sauce
Wasabi
1 tbsp (6 g) thinly sliced scallions
Thinly sliced lemon
Hot sauce

THE METHOD

Make the cauliflower rice by placing the florets in a food processor; pulse until their texture is like rice. Add the vinegar and lemon juice and mix the ingredients together by hand. Set the the mixture aside.

To prep the tomato tuna, bring a small pot of water to a boil. Also grab a bowl of ice with some water in it for an ice bath. Core your tomatoes from the top and pop them in the water for 2 minutes until the skin starts to peel off. With a slotted spoon, transfer the tomatoes to the ice bath. Once cool, remove the skin with a pairing knife, cut in half and remove the inside with the seeds so all that's left is the meaty shell part of the tomatoes. Slice into 1-inch (2.5-cm) slices and place in a bowl. In a Mason jar, add sesame oil, liquid aminos, coconut aminos and vinegar and mix well. Pour over the tomatoes and marinate for 30 minutes.

Next, prep your rolls. I like to arrange the cucumber, avocado, mango, tomato tuna and radish on a plate for easy access. Place a sushi mat on a clean, flat surface. Place a small bowl of water next to the mat. Place 1 nori sheet on the mat rough side up. Place a thin layer of the cauliflower rice on top of the nori, leaving about 1 inch (2.5 cm) of space around the sides. Press down with your fingers, so that the rice is nice and tight.

Place a few slices of avocado horizontally in a line on the very bottom of the nori sheet. Then add the cucumber, mango, tomato and radish, making horizontal layers and building upward. Once the layers of veggies are assembled, lift up the bottom edge of the sushi mat and fold over the fillings until they are inside the roll, still leaving 1 inch (2.5 cm) of the empty nori sheet exposed on the top. Use the sushi mat to help you pinch the sushi roll together, and press and hold it for a few seconds. Dip your finger in the bowl of water and dampen the exposed nori, then finish rolling the sushi until it's tightly wrapped. Moisten a very sharp knife with water and quickly slice the sushi roll into individual pieces.

Repeat for each roll, making sure your knife is moist and clean between cuts. Serve the sushi with the garnishes of your choice.

Makes 4 sushi rolls

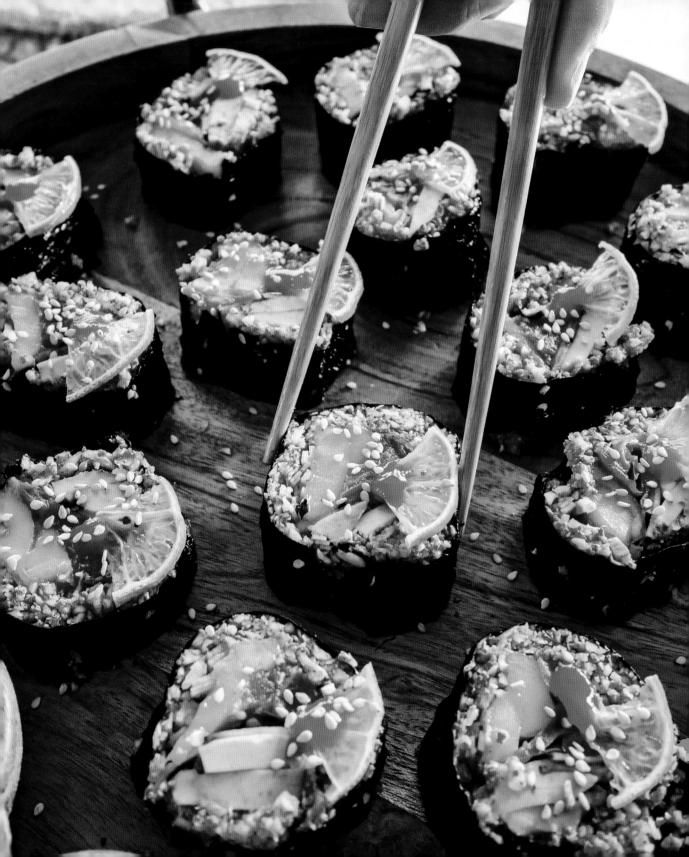

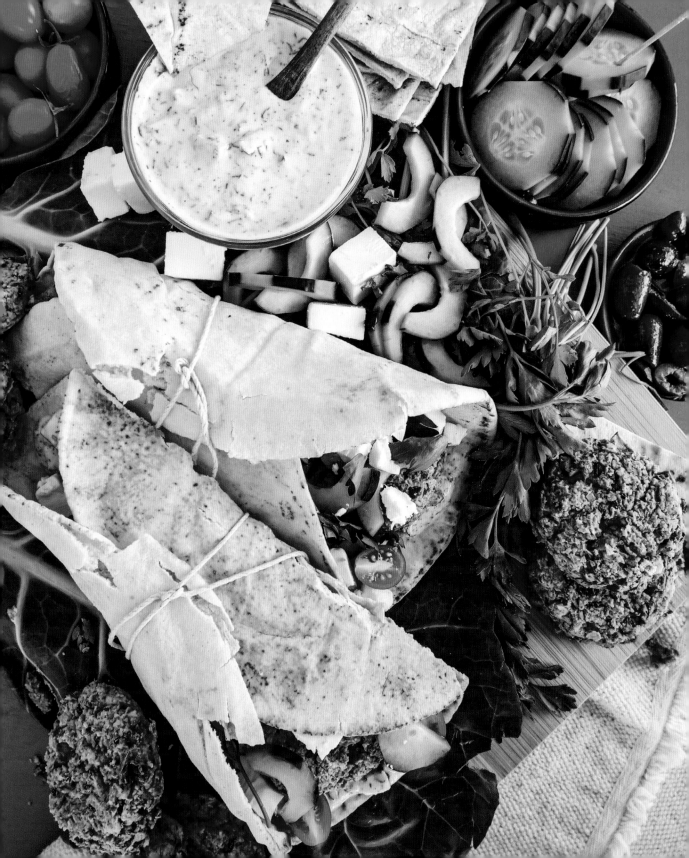

FALAFEL WRAPS WITH TZATZIKI SAUCE

Falafel is the most epic way to get Mediterranean flavor, plant-based protein and a to-go meal all in one. When you're switching to a plant-based diet, falafel are great for meal prep—they keep well in the freezer for those super busy workdays, and they work well as your protein on top of a salad. Any way you look at it, falafel will always be there for you. My husband, Steve, is the falafel master, and I owe this oil-free recipe to him. Our secret ingredient is black beans, as they create an amazing texture and flavor. These baked falafel are paired perfectly with our creamy tzatziki.

THE GOODS

FALAFEL

1 (15-oz [425-g]) can black beans, drained and rinsed

1 (15-oz [425-g]) can garbanzo beans, drained and rinsed

½ medium red onion, diced

3 tbsp (45 ml) fresh lemon juice

¼ cup (60 g) tahini

4 cloves garlic, minced

1 tsp salt

½ tsp black pepper

1 tsp ground cumin

¾ cup (72 g) almond flour

½ packed cup (60 g) fresh parsley, minced

1 heaping tbsp (20 g) capers, undrained

2 tbsp (20 g) pepperoncini, diced

TZATZIKI SAUCE

1 cup (240 ml) Cashew Cream (page 173) or plain coconut yogurt

¼ cup (12 g) chopped parsley

¼ cup (12 g) chopped fresh mint

¼ cup (60 ml) fresh lemon juice

1 cup (133 g) chopped cucumber

½ tsp granulated garlic or 3 cloves garlic, minced

½ tsp salt

½ tsp black pepper

WRAPS

4 large pita breads

15 cherry tomatoes, cut in half

½ medium cucumber, sliced

1 block Herbed Creamy Feta (page 166), crumbled

THE METHOD

To make the falafel, preheat the oven to 375°F (191°C). Line a large baking sheet with parchment paper.

In a large bowl, combine the black beans, garbanzo beans, onion, lemon juice, tahini, garlic, salt, black pepper, cumin, flour, parsley, capers and their juice and pepperoncini. Mash the ingredients with a potato masher or process in a food processor until the mixture starts to stick together. I don't like it to be fully pureed, as I enjoy seeing the contrast between the colorful ingredients.

Scoop out lime-sized balls of the falafel mixture and place them on the prepared baking sheet. Press down lightly to make them flat disks. I use the bottom of a glass and twist it while I press and release. Bake the falafel for 30 minutes, until they are starting to turn golden brown.

Meanwhile, make your tzatziki sauce. In a medium bowl, stir together the Cashew Cream, parsley, mint, lemon juice, cucumber, granulated garlic, salt and black pepper. Voilà! If you're not making the wraps right away, store the tzatziki, covered, in the fridge.

To assemble your wraps, heat the pita breads over an open flame on the stove for 3 to 5 seconds on each side. Alternatively, you can warm them on a medium baking sheet in the oven at 350°F (177°C) for 3 to 5 minutes.

Spread about ¼ cup (60 ml) of the tzatziki on the bottom-middle portion of each pita, then add two or three falafel to the bottom portion. Add a few cherry tomatoes, a few cucumber slices and some Herbed Creamy Feta. Wrap each pita by folding the sides over—you can tie the wrap with twine if it won't stay together. Serve the wraps immediately or make them ahead of time to take with you. We love taking these wraps to the beach for the perfect picnic!

Makes 4 wraps

RUSTIC ITALIAN CHOPPED SALAD

Chopped salads are especially good for lunch, as they have all you need to feel totally satisfied and make you feel like you did something great for your body. I love a good chopped salad at my favorite Italian restaurant with a big ol' bowl of pasta and a glorious glass of Sangiovese. Regardless of whether you're channeling this Italian pasta night to your workday or you are cookin' up something special for a date night, this salad will hit the spot. The dressing is one you should have in your toolbox to whip out at the last minute, as it's delicious on almost anything. This classic salad is perfect as a Mason jar lunch, because it travels well and, once you dump it in a bowl, you've got yourself the most epic on-the-go meal. Rustic Italian never tasted so good.

THE GOODS

DRESSING

3 tbsp (45 ml) olive oil

2 tbsp (30 ml) red wine vinegar

2 tsp (10 g) Dijon mustard

1 tbsp (15 ml) pure maple syrup

1 tbsp (15 ml) fresh lemon juice

¼ tsp salt

¼ tsp black pepper

SALAD

1 cup (90 g) finely chopped purple cabbage

1 cup (150 g) cherry tomatoes, thinly sliced

1 (15-oz [425-g]) can cannellini or great northern beans, drained and rinsed

½ cup (70 g) thinly sliced black olives

½ medium cucumber, coarsely chopped

¼ cup (14 g) bagged or jarred sun-dried tomatoes

1 cup (170 g) marinated quartered artichoke hearts, drained

½ cup (80 g) pepperoncini, thinly sliced

¼ cup (45 g) crumbled Herbed Creamy Feta (page 166)

2 tbsp (30 g) capers, drained

1 medium bunch kale, destemmed and thinly sliced (see Bai's Tip)

THE METHOD

First, make your dressing. In a medium bowl or Mason jar, mix together the oil, vinegar, mustard, maple syrup, lemon juice, salt and black pepper.

To prep the salad in Mason jars, grab three or four 32-ounce (907-g) jars and distribute the dressing evenly in of the bottoms of the jars. Next, place the cabbage on top of the dressing evenly. Layer the cherry tomatoes, beans, olives, cucumber, sun-dried tomatoes, artichoke hearts, pepperoncini, Herbed Creamy Feta, capers and kale on the cabbage. Secure the lids on the jars and place the salads in the fridge. The salads will keep in the fridge really well for 5 to 7 days.

If you are making a large family-style salad, mix together the cabbage, cherry tomatoes, beans, olives, cucumber, sun-dried tomatoes, artichoke hearts, pepperoncini, Herbed Creamy Feta, capers and kale in a large salad bowl. I like the ingredients to be combined, but you can also layer the salad with the greens first and then assemble the toppings in whatever way you'd like. Toss the salad with the dressing and serve it immediately.

BAI'S TIP: If you aren't a huge kale fan, feel free to use your favorite lettuce for this recipe, as they all go great with it!

Makes 3 to 4 servings

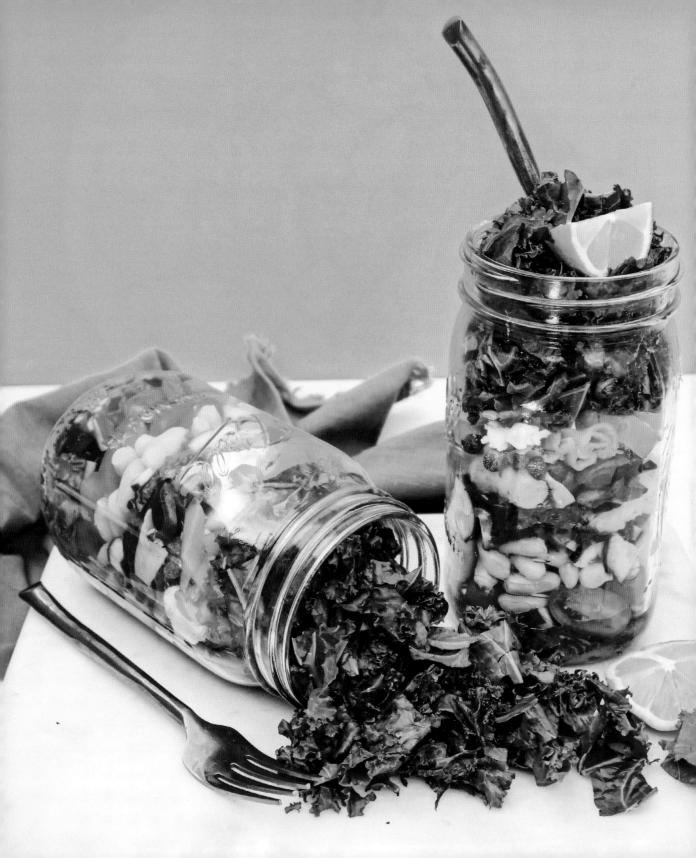

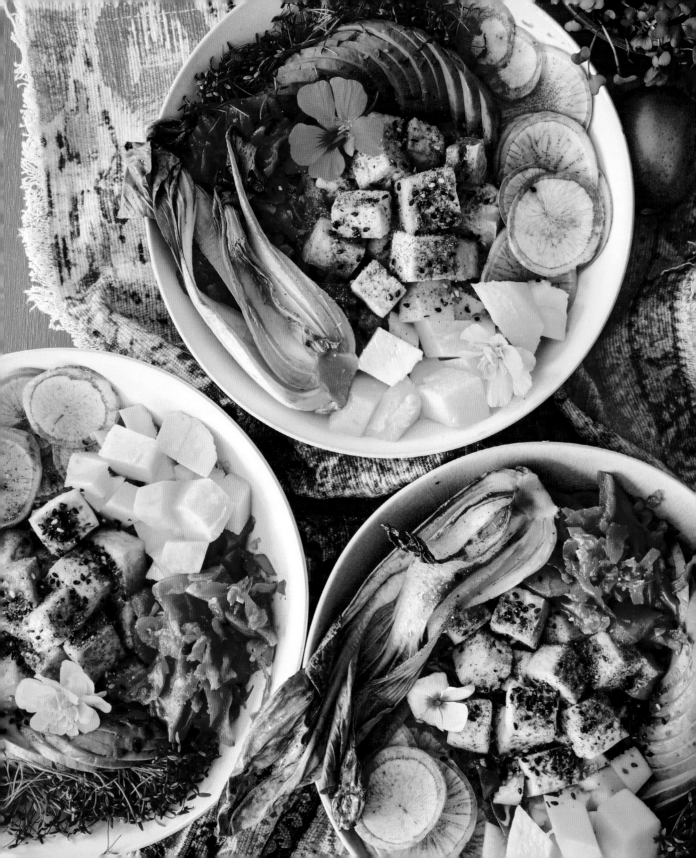

CRISPY TOFU RAINBOW BALI BOWL

Bali, Indonesia, is a mecca for healing. Visiting that island changed my life and sped up my physical and emotional healing process. The energy is less rushed, daily actions are fueled with intention and, well, the food is some of the best plant-based food I've ever had. This rainbow bowl contains the bright yet humble energy that Bali possesses. This recipe uses such simple ingredients and concepts, but when they are all put together, the result is delicious and healing. Make this as a meal prep or as a delish lunch with friends. It will bring you lots of plant protein, colorful food and good energy.

THE GOODS

BOWLS

1 cup (200 g) quinoa, rinsed

1½ cups (360 ml) Immune-Boosting Veggie Broth (page 170)

1 (14-oz [397-g]) block firm tofu, drained and pressed (see Bai's Tips)

1 tsp salt (optional)

2 tbsp (30 ml) coconut aminos

2 medium bunches bok choy, cut in half

¼ large head cabbage, thinly sliced

1 small watermelon or red radish, thinly sliced

2 medium avocados, thinly sliced

¼ cup (60 g) vegan kimchi or sauerkraut, drained

½ cup (83 g) diced mango

DRESSING

2 tbsp (30 ml) toasted sesame oil

2 tbsp (30 ml) coconut aminos

2 tbsp (30 ml) plain rice vinegar

2 tbsp (30 ml) fresh lime juice

GARNISHES

Sesame seeds

Micro greens

Edible flowers (optional)

THE METHOD

In a small saucepan over medium-high heat, combine the quinoa and broth. Bring to a boil, reduce the heat to low, cover the saucepan and simmer the quinoa for 18 minutes, until the broth has been absorbed. Let the quinoa rest, covered, while you continue making the bowls.

Meanwhile, preheat your oven to 350°F (177°C). Line a large baking sheet with parchment paper.

Cut the tofu into ½-inch (1.3-cm) cubes. Place the tofu cubes on the prepared baking sheet. They'll be crispy, high-protein croutons for your bowl, so there is no need to season them unless you would like to add the optional salt. Bake the tofu for 30 minutes, tossing the cubes halfway through the baking time, until they are crispy.

While the quinoa and the tofu are doing their thing, pour the coconut aminos in a shallow bowl and dip each side of the four pieces of bok choy in the bowl to coat them with the coconut aminos. Heat a medium cast-iron or stainless steel skillet over medium-high heat—do not use a nonstick skillet. Sear the bok choy for 1 to 2 minutes on each side, until it is starting to turn golden brown. Set aside.

Prep your dressing. In a jar, combine the oil, coconut aminos, vinegar and lime juice. Secure the jar's lid and shake until the dressing is smooth. Set aside.

Now it's time to build the bowls. First, place a hefty scoop of quinoa in the bottom of three bowls. Top it with the cabbage, tofu, bok choy, radish, avocado, kimchi and mango. Drizzle the dressing over the top of each serving. Garnish each serving with the sesame seeds, micro greens and edible flowers (if using).

BAI'S TIP: Press the tofu by draining it and then drying it off in a clean kitchen towel. Wrap it in the towel and place something somewhat heavy on top, like a carton of veggie broth or a baking dish, and let the tofu press for 20 minutes.

Makes 3 bowls

THE REUBEN

There was an entire year when my husband and I went on a search for the absolute best vegan Reuben. We went to Chicago, San Francisco, Denver, Los Angeles and even Bali. The two sandwiches that topped them all were from The Chicago Diner and Peloton Supershop in Bali. The thing that made these Reubens stand out? The high quality of the bread, the overall simplicity of the recipes and the dedication to the classic flavors of the Reuben. When you think of going vegan, usually the idea of enjoying a Reuben again seems unlikely. I'm here to tell you that it's possible. The key? Don't skimp on the bread! Use one with a crispy crust and a soft interior, like the Seeded Herbed Spelt Bread on page 178.

THE GOODS

MARINATED TEMPEH

¼ cup (60 ml) vegan Worcestershire sauce

1 tbsp (15 ml) liquid smoke

½ tsp granulated garlic

½ tsp smoked paprika

½ tsp mustard powder

¼ tsp horseradish

2 tsp (10 ml) pure maple syrup

1 tbsp (15 ml) Immune-Boosting Veggie Broth (page 170) or water

8 oz (227 g) plain tempeh

THOUSAND ISLAND DRESSING

¼ cup (60 ml) Cashew Cream (page 173) or vegan mayo

2 tsp (16 g) tomato paste

1 tbsp (15 g) sweet relish

1 medium white onion, minced

½ tsp horseradish

¼ tsp salt

½ tsp Dijon mustard

1 tsp pure maple syrup

SANDWICHES

4 slices rye, sourdough or gluten-free bread

Not Your Mama's Salted Butter (page 158) or store-bought vegan butter, as needed (optional)

2 slices vegan Swiss, Gouda or provolone cheese

1 cup (240 g) red sauerkraut

THE METHOD

First, prep the marinated tempeh. In a small jar, combine the Worcestershire sauce, liquid smoke, granulated garlic, smoked paprika, mustard powder, horseradish, maple syrup and broth. Secure the jar's lid and shake it for 15 seconds to create the marinade. Cut the tempeh in half lengthwise, so that you have two thin, long pieces. Then slice each one into three, so that you have a total of six pieces. Place the tempeh in a medium baking dish and pour the marinade over the top. Place the baking dish in the fridge and let the tempeh marinate for at least 30 minutes. This would be great to prep the day before and marinate overnight.

While your tempeh is doin' its thing, make the Thousand Island dressing. In a medium bowl, stir together the Cashew Cream, tomato paste, relish, onion, horseradish, salt, Dijon mustard and maple syrup. Make sure the dressing is smooth.

When you're ready to build the sandwiches, toast the bread in a toaster or in a hot skillet with a little butter. While it's toasting, heat a medium skillet over medium-high heat. Add the tempeh and sear each side for 2 minutes, until the tempeh is golden brown. I like to pour the marinade over the tempeh while it's searing to add extra flavor.

On 2 slices of the bread, layer the tempeh, Swiss cheese, sauerkraut and Thousand Island dressing. Top the sandwiches with the remaining 2 slices of bread. Cut each sandwich in half, then transfer both sandwiches to two serving plates. Serve right away. You'll definitely need a napkin for this one!

BAI'S TIP: Eat this sandwich when it's hot. I even recommend placing it on a baking sheet and popping it into the oven at 400°F (204°C) for 5 to 7 minutes right before you eat it, if you're feeling like going the extra mile.

Makes 2 sandwiches

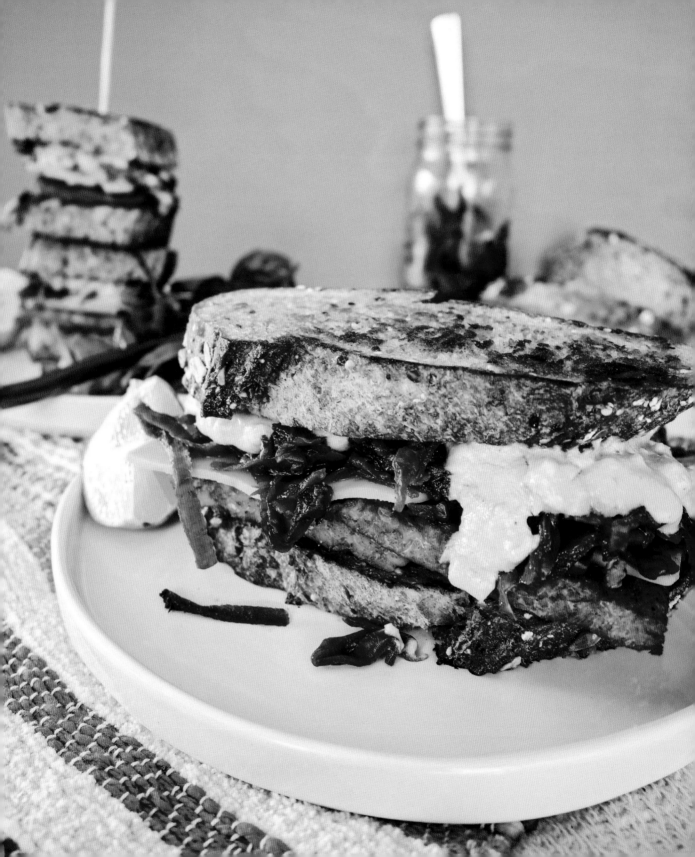

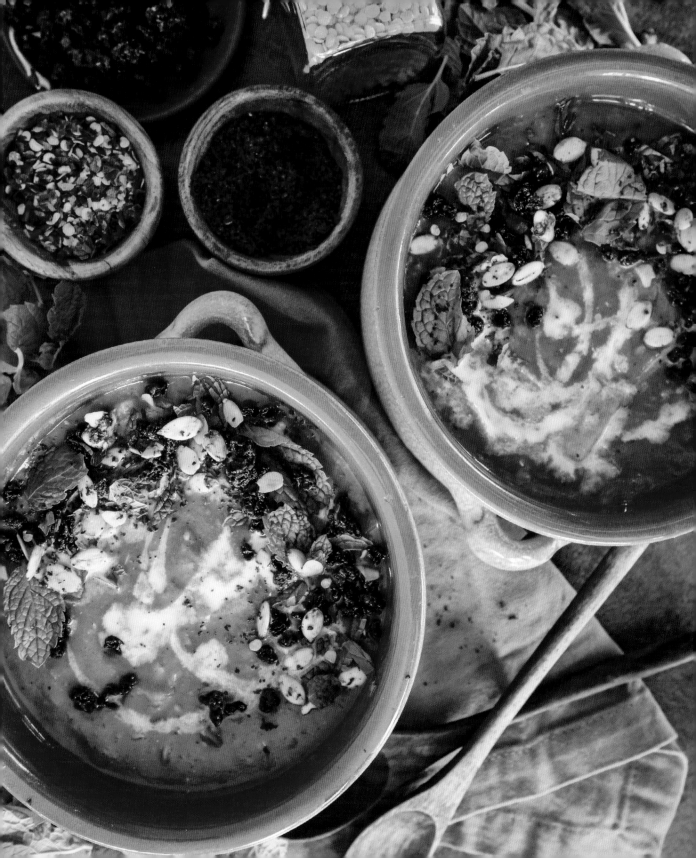

MOROCCAN LENTIL SOUP

Everyone needs a go-to soup when they're feeling under the weather, and this is mine. In fact, this is one of the first recipes I taught my husband to make when we were dating, as it's the ultimate comforting, warmly spiced dish to make you feel better. Lentil soup is a great entry-level food when you're starting out with this whole vegan thing. It's naturally plant-based, and this Moroccan twist will make you feel like you're a pro already. The chopped mint, dried currants, cinnamon and sumac give this traditional Middle Eastern soup seriously deep flavor without overcomplicating things. Move over, chicken noodle—there's a new favorite in town!

THE GOODS

SOUP
1 tsp olive oil
1 medium onion, finely chopped
Pinch plus 2 tsp (10 g) of salt, divided
1½ cups (120 g) finely chopped leeks
1 cup (100 g) finely chopped fennel
2 medium ribs celery, finely chopped
1 large carrot, finely chopped
½ tsp black pepper
1 tsp mustard seeds
1 tsp ground cinnamon
1 tsp ground coriander
½ tsp ground ginger
4 cups (960 ml) Immune-Boosting Veggie Broth (page 170), divided
2 medium red potatoes, diced into small pieces
1 medium sweet potato, diced into small pieces
¾ cup (150 g) red lentils, rinsed
1 cup (240 ml) coconut milk
1 tsp sumac or za'atar (see Bai's Tip)

GARNISHES
Dried currants
Finely chopped fresh mint
Roasted salted pumpkin seeds

THE METHOD

To make the soup, heat the oil in a large pot over medium-high heat. Add the onion and the pinch of salt. Cook the onion for 2 to 3 minutes, until it is soft and fragrant. Add the leeks and fennel and cook the vegetables for about 2 minutes, until some of the goods are starting to toast and turn golden brown. Add the celery, carrot, black pepper, 1 teaspoon of the salt, mustard seeds, cinnamon, coriander and ginger. Stir to coat all the veggies in the spices. Sauté the mixture for 2 to 3 minutes. You'll notice a buildup of spices on the bottom of the pot at this point, so add a splash of the broth to deglaze the pot. Add the red potatoes, sweet potato and lentils. Toast everything for 2 to 3 minutes. Again, if the mixture starts to build up on the bottom of the pot, add a splash of the broth.

Add the remaining broth, cover the pot, reduce the heat to medium-low and cook the soup for 15 to 20 minutes, stirring it occasionally, until the lentils and veggies are tender. Uncover the pot and add the milk, sumac and remaining 1 teaspoon of salt.

Transfer half of the soup to a blender. Blend the soup until it's creamy. Pour the blended soup into the pot to create a thick and luscious soup. If you prefer the soup chunky and brothy, skip the blending.

Ladle the desired amount of soup into four or five soup bowls. Top each serving with the currants, mint and pumpkin seeds.

BAI'S TIP: If you choose to use za'atar, make sure it includes sumac.

Makes 4 to 5 servings

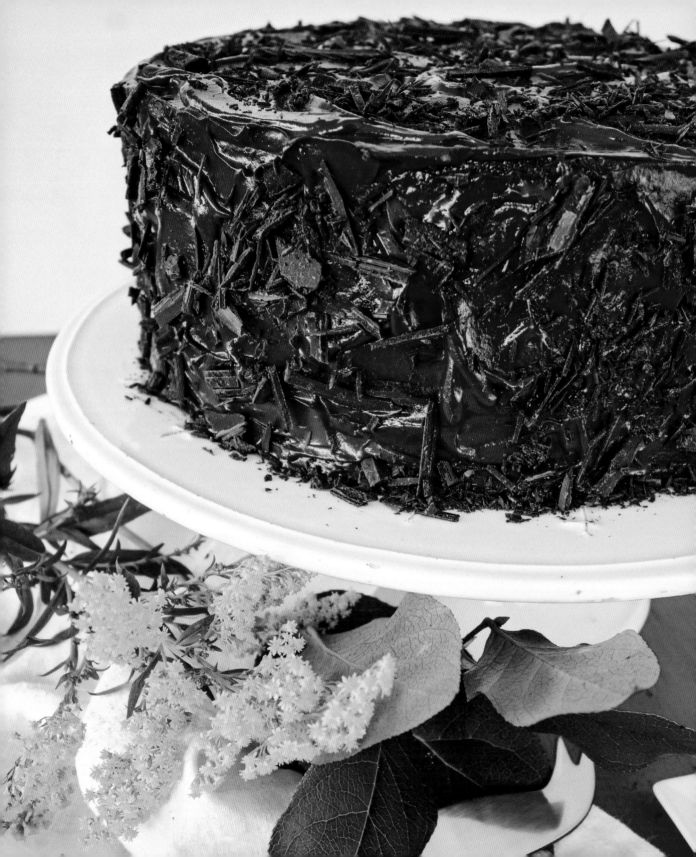

A HEALTHY *Sweet Tooth*

Let's start normalizing saying yes to pleasure as part of a healthy diet and lifestyle. There's a common misconception that you lose the aspect of eating for pleasure when switching to a plant-based diet. Nothing could be further from the truth! What you do lose is the idea of a "guilty" pleasure. You are able to fully step into unapologetically doing things for you.

Finding your ultimate pleasure through food is the secret sauce to happiness and freedom within yourself. What we eat and how we eat is a reflection of how we feel about ourselves and how we allow ourselves to truly be satisfied. Not on a level that stops at our mouth when we eat something, but at a level that affects every single cell of our bodies. Truly being satisfied isn't surface level; it will last for hours after your meal. And that is exactly what we're after.

I got my first job when I was eleven, working in a pastry kitchen. I mainly set up cake boxes, filled cannoli and dunked strawberries in chocolate. Don't worry, it wasn't a child-labor issue—I actually begged my mom to let me work for this pastry chef instead of going to summer camp. I found the whole process of making desserts totally mind-blowing. Melting chocolate, cutting fruit, smelling a cake as it bakes: It's the whole experience that can hit all of our pleasure centers. There is a reason kids love cookies so much—they are such a simple way to experience joy unapologetically.

This chapter is a way to celebrate our life in the most delicious and delectable way. It's also a way to celebrate by being kind to our bodies, our planet and the animals that live on it. I believe that to truly tap into celebration and joy, we have to do it in a way that respects the world around us. Pastries can be made with butter made from plants; cookies can be made without refined sugar, eggs and refined flour; and cheesecake can be just as decadent without harming any cows in the process.

At first, baking totally vegan feels like a tall order, and I'll admit it's not easy at first, especially when creating your own recipes. Add a gluten-free aspect to that and, well, you've got yourself a major project! I took care of the hard part and created these easy-to-follow recipes to help you tap into your pleasure center and unapologetically find joy in your kitchen.

DARK CHOCOLATE OATMEAL COOKIE SKILLET

For kids, there is a sense of accomplishment, the pleasure of satisfied cravings and the feeling of sheer happiness that comes with learning how to make cookies and eating them fresh from the oven. Honestly, I owe my love for cooking and my keen sense of timing to my early baking days. This cookie skillet recipe is dedicated to the inner child that resides within all of us! Since it's totally gluten-free, refined sugar-free and made from plants, you can rest easy knowing that this recipe will take care of you—and your inner child too.

THE GOODS

2 tbsp (12 g) ground chia seeds

¼ cup (60 ml) plus 1 tbsp (15 ml) water

½ cup (120 g) smooth almond butter

¾ cup (120 g) coconut sugar

¼ cup (60 ml) melted coconut oil or Not Your Mama's Salted Butter (page 158), plus more as needed

¼ cup (60 ml) cashew milk or plant milk of choice

1 tsp pure vanilla extract

1¼ cups (120 g) almond flour

½ tsp baking soda

1 cup (90 g) rolled oats

1 (3-oz [85-g]) vegan dark chocolate bar, broken into pieces

½ tsp flaky sea salt

Vegan vanilla ice cream, for serving

THE METHOD

Preheat your oven to 350°F (177°C).

In a large bowl, make two chia eggs by mixing together the ground chia seeds and water. Let the mixture sit and thicken for 1 minute. Once the chia has absorbed all the water, add the almond butter, sugar, oil, milk and vanilla. Mix the ingredients well with a spatula or wooden spoon.

In a medium bowl, mix together the almond flour and baking soda with a fork. Make sure to break up any clumps of baking soda. Add the almond flour mixture to the chia mixture. Next, fold in the oats.

Evenly coat a 10-inch (25-cm) ovenproof skillet with additional oil. If you want to avoid oil for this step, you can line with parchment paper instead. Add the cookie dough to the skillet and press down so it's nice and even. Top the cookie with the chocolate pieces and sprinkle the sea salt on top.

Bake the cookie for 25 to 30 minutes, until it is golden brown. It'll lift easily from around the side of the skillet and will still be soft to the touch in the middle. Remove the cookie from the oven and let it cool for at least 10 minutes. Top it with vegan ice cream and dive right in.

BAI'S TIP: Make individual cookies with this same recipe! Just scoop balls out onto a baking sheet 2 inches (5 cm) apart and bake the cookies for 8 to 10 minutes.

Makes 1 (10-inch [25-cm]) cookie

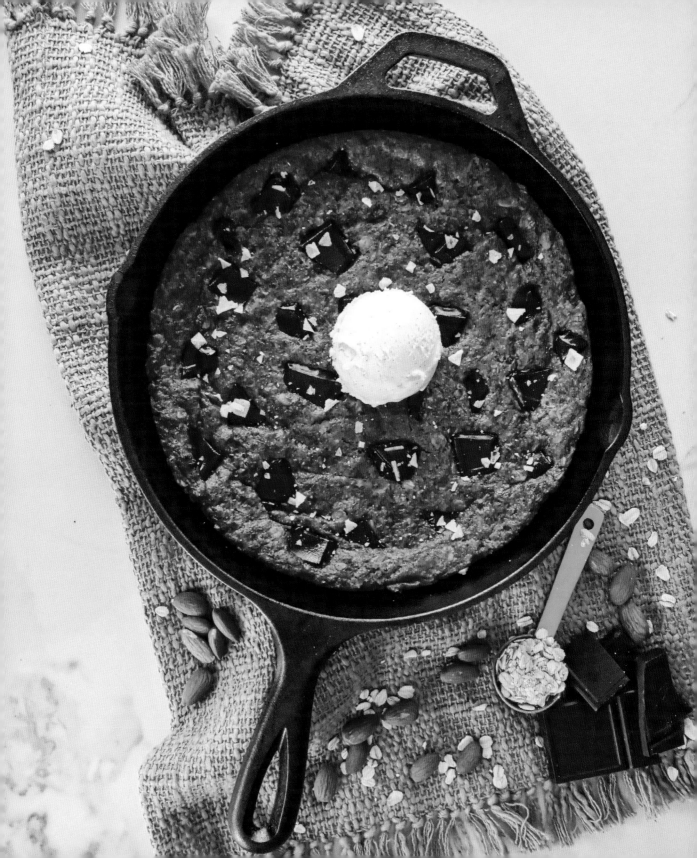

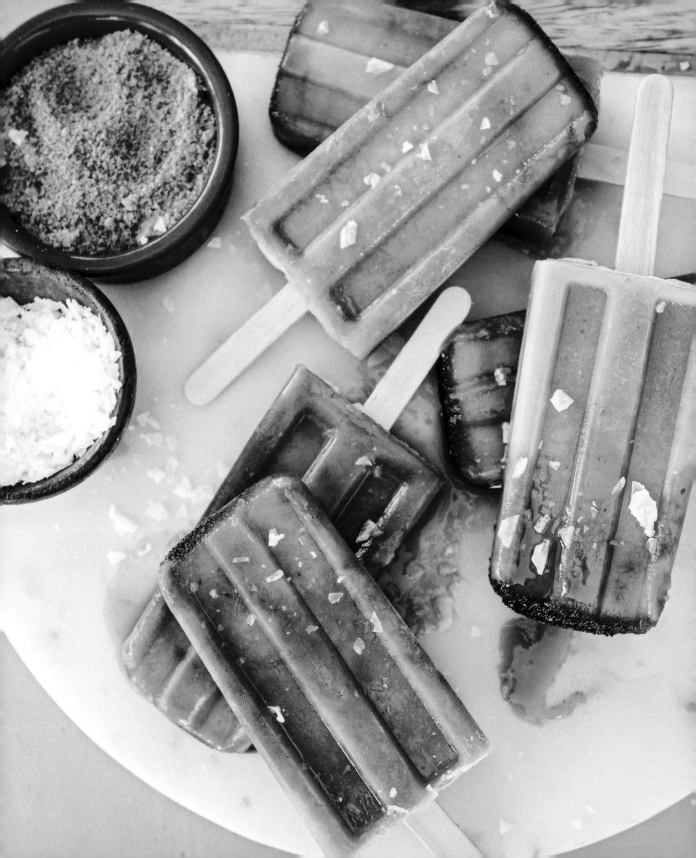

SALTED DULCE DE LECHE POPS

Mmmm! Dulce de leche is so smooth, creamy and sweet—everything you'd want and more from a dessert. Traditional dulce de leche is from Argentina, and it's created with milk and sugar. Essentially, it's a next-level caramel sauce that pairs beautifully with almost everything. This was the inspiration for these pops. They're made from creamy cashew milk and coconut sugar, two healthy alternatives to the classic dulce de leche. Because this recipe is salted, these popsicles hit the spot all year-round. Not only do they cool you down on a hot day but they also vibe with you during the holidays. Plant-based custard ice cream covered with dulce de leche on a stick will quickly become your new favorite way to satisfy your sweet tooth.

THE GOODS

2½ cups (600 ml) Cashew-Hemp Milk (page 162)

½ cup (80 g) coconut sugar, divided

½ tsp pure vanilla extract

2 tbsp (18 g) tapioca flour

¼ cup (60 ml) water

½ tsp flaky sea salt

THE METHOD

In a small saucepan, combine the milk, ¼ cup (40 g) of the sugar, vanilla and tapioca flour. Turn the heat to medium-high and cook the mixture for 3 to 4 minutes, stirring it frequently. Once the consistency begins to thicken at about 3 minutes, remove the saucepan from the heat and set it aside. This will be the frozen custard that makes this recipe so good.

In another small saucepan over medium-high heat, combine the remaining ¼ cup (40 g) sugar, water and sea salt. Stir the mixture constantly with a rubber spatula for about 2 minutes. The sugar will dissolve to create the caramel sauce. It will still be watery and not fully caramelized yet. Remove the saucepan from the heat. Let both mixtures cool for 5 to 10 minutes.

Grab an ice pop mold and fill each mold with about ½ inch (1.3 cm) of the caramel sauce, just to create the tips of the pops. Sprinkle a few flakes of the sea salt over the caramel sauce, then finish filling the molds with the custard mixture. Cover the ice pop mold with the lid and place wooden ice pop handles in the pops. Freeze the pops for at least 6 hours, or overnight.

Once they are frozen, run the mold under hot water for 10 seconds to remove the pops more easily.

Makes 8 to 9 pops

PECAN-CACAO DATE BARS

This is not just another granola bar. Though there are a million options out there, these bars have no refined sugar—rather, they're made with simple ingredients and goods that'll give you real, lasting energy. This is my ideal granola bar that also works great as a late-night chocolate snack. Dates hold these bars together and, in a way, they can help hold us together too: They've got loads of iron, are rich in vitamins, can help lower cholesterol, are supporters of clear skin and are an amazing natural sweetener. Talk about the ideal superfood! Match the dates with cacao and pecans and you've got yourself a serious mood booster.

THE GOODS

2 cups (200 g) pecans

½ cup (56 g) cacao powder

1½ cups (210 g) pitted Medjool dates

2 tbsp (12 g) ground chia seeds

¼ cup (23 g) rolled oats

1 tbsp (15 ml) melted coconut oil

¼ tsp salt

THE METHOD

In a food processor, combine the pecans, cacao, dates, ground chia seeds, oats, oil and salt. Process the ingredients on low speed for 2 to 3 minutes. You should be able to easily form the mixture into a firm ball.

Grab a 9 x 9-inch (23 x 23-cm) baking pan and line it with parchment paper. Dump the mixture in the prepared baking pan, and then press down on the mixture with another sheet of parchment paper to make it tight and even. Refrigerate the mixture for 30 minutes. Once it has chilled, cut it into squares and keep the bars in an airtight container or silicone bag in your fridge. Enjoy them on the go, after a workout or on your favorite hiking trail!

Makes 16 square bars

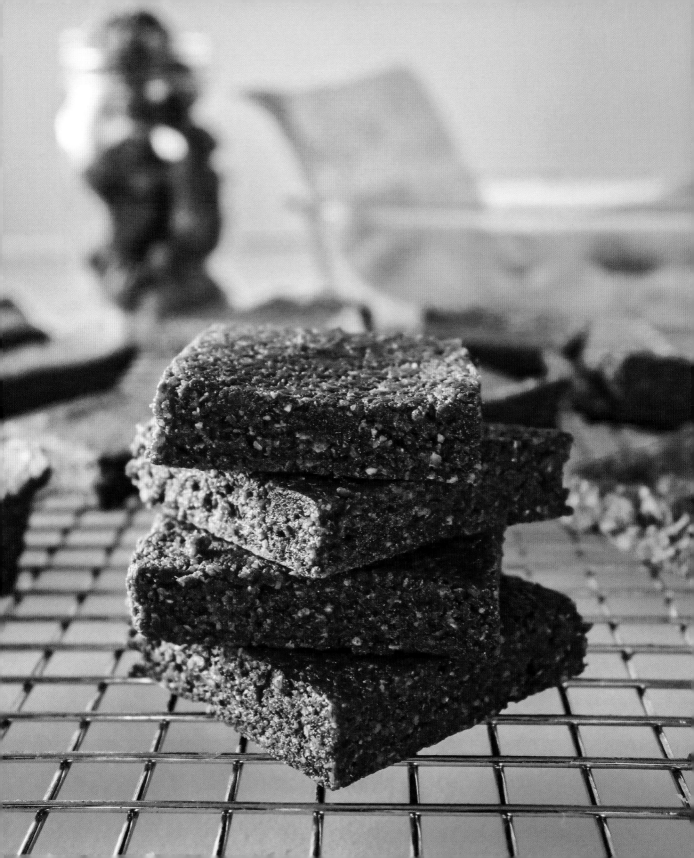

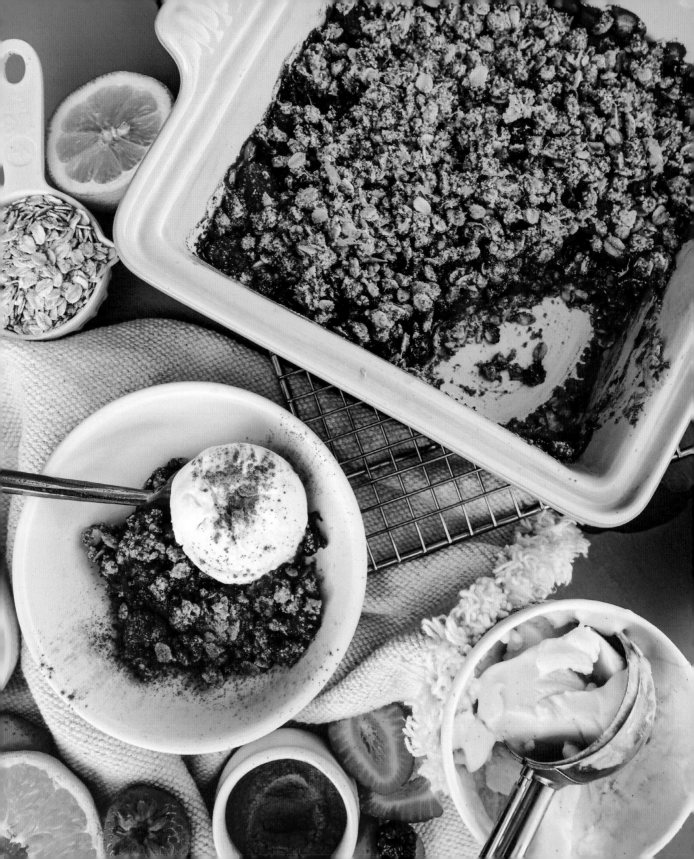

BERRY CRUMBLE

Although I am a chocoholic by nature, my heart always has room for a fruit-forward dessert like this one. My inner lazy girl loves a good crumble, as I feel it's the simplified way to make a pie without the fuss of making a crust. A really good crumble is perfectly sweet and crumbly while still giving you all those pie feels. A traditional crumble is easily veganized by swapping butter for coconut oil. If you aren't into the coconut flavor of coconut oil, be sure to get refined coconut oil, as it's flavorless. This crumble pairs so epically with vegan vanilla ice cream, you'll have a hard time not keeping this one for yourself!

THE GOODS

1½ cups (144 g) almond flour

1 cup (90 g) rolled oats

½ cup (80 g) coconut sugar

1 tsp ground cinnamon

½ cup (120 g) cold coconut oil

½ tsp salt

3 cups (399 g) fresh or frozen mixed berries (such as cherries, blackberries, blueberries and raspberries)

1 tbsp (15 ml) fresh orange juice

1 tbsp (15 ml) fresh lemon juice

3 tbsp (27 g) tapioca flour

1 tbsp (15 ml) pure maple syrup

Vegan vanilla ice cream, for serving

THE METHOD

Preheat the oven to 350°F (177°C).

In a large bowl, combine the almond flour, oats, sugar, cinnamon, oil and salt. Stir the ingredients with a spoon or with your hands until they are well combined. Set the mixture aside.

In a medium bowl, combine the berries, orange juice, lemon juice, tapioca flour and maple syrup. Mix until the berries are evenly coated and the tapioca flour is absorbed by the citrus juices.

Grab a 9 x 9-inch (23 x 23-cm) baking dish and add three-fourths of the crumble mixture to the bottom. Press down firmly on the crumble. Add the berry goodness on top. Once you have evenly distributed your berry mixture over the crumble, sprinkle the remaining one-fourth of the crumble over the top of the berries. Bake the crumble for 30 minutes, until the berry sauce is bubbling and the top is golden brown. Serve the crumble warm with the vanilla ice cream and good vibes.

Makes 1 (9 x 9-inch [23 x 23-cm]) crumble

PISTACHIO, CHERRY AND CACAO NO-CHURN ICE CREAM

This is a flavor combo that I just fell into one day a few years ago, thanks to my stocked pantry—I have been making it ever since. Basically, it's the best accident ever! In our house, my husband and I are really serious about ice cream—my husband actually has a tattoo of an ice cream cone. So when we decided to make our own, we knew it was going to be epic. The pistachios add the body and creaminess, the cherries round out the nuttiness with their sweet tartness and the cacao . . . I mean, need I say more? With bananas as the base, this is an ideal low-sugar, whole-food, raw recipe that is perfect for getting kids to try new things and getting my husband to eat less refined sugar. No matter the crowd, they'll be sure to ask for this one again and again!

THE GOODS

3 medium ripe peeled and frozen bananas

1½ heaping cups (230 g) frozen cherries, plus more as needed

½ cup (120 ml) Cashew-Hemp Milk (page 162) or plant milk of choice

1 tbsp (15 ml) pure maple syrup

3 tbsp (21 g) cacao powder

¼ cup (40 g) raw shelled pistachios, plus more as needed

½ cup (85 g) vegan dark chocolate chips, plus more as needed

THE METHOD

In a high-powered blender or food processor, combine the bananas, cherries, milk, maple syrup, cacao and pistachios. Blend the ingredients on high speed until they are smooth.

Add the chocolate chips and blend for 5 to 10 seconds to slightly break them up and distribute them throughout the ice cream. Pour the ice cream into a freezer-safe 1-quart (946-ml) dish. Spread the ice cream out evenly in the dish. Freeze the ice cream for 15 minutes.

Scoop it into bowls and top each serving with extra cherries, pistachios and chocolate chips. Or enjoy the ice cream in a cone!

Makes 1 quart (946 ml)

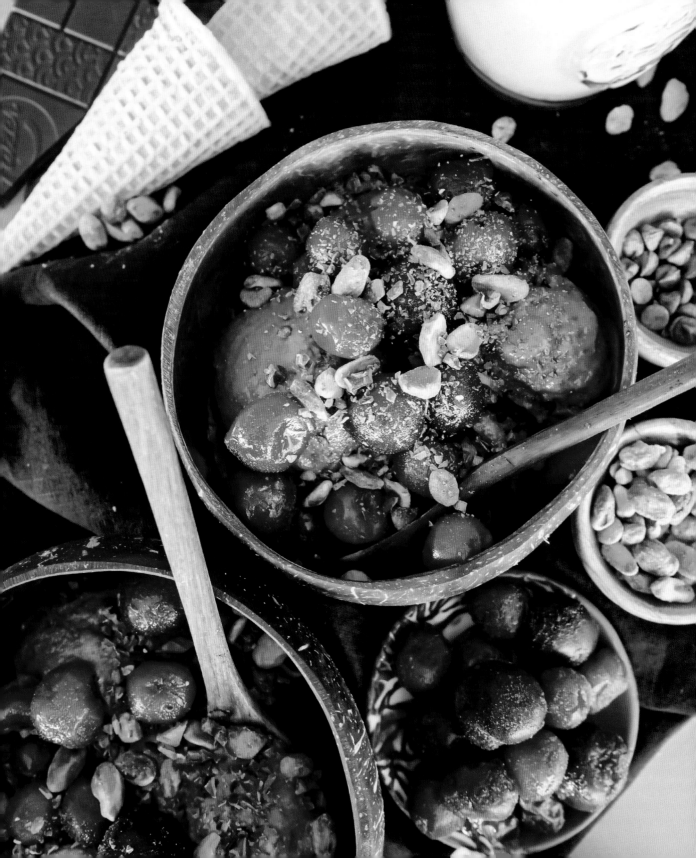

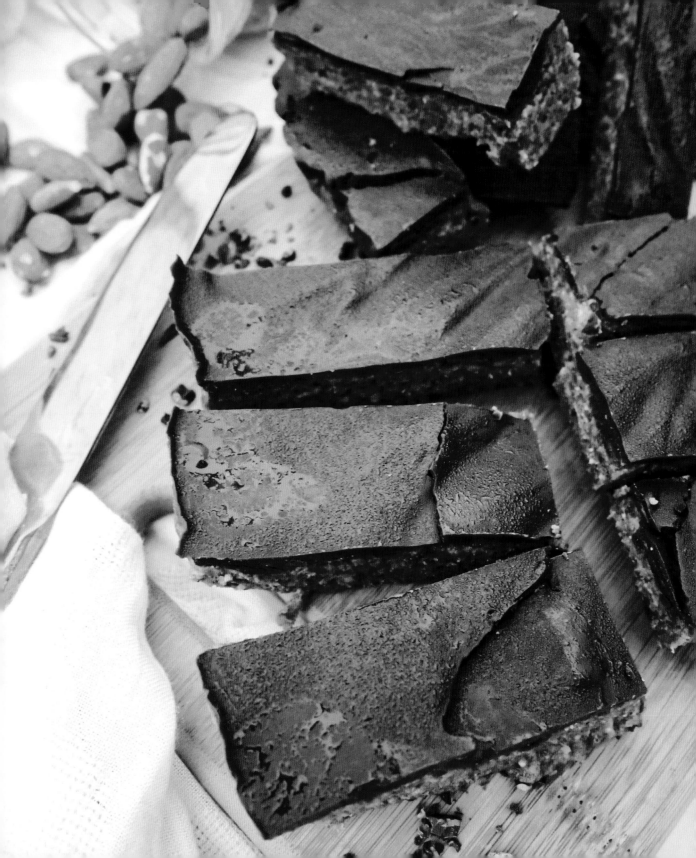

CHAI-SPICED ALMOND CHOCOLATE BARS

I'll take chai-spiced everything, please! There is a reason why chai-spiced food is so freakin'
delicious. The spices not only enliven our taste buds, but also they enliven every cell in our bodies.
Spices have the ability to lower blood sugar, fight inflammation, keep your heart healthy, ease
nausea and relieve pain—they even have cancer-fighting compounds. They are incredibly potent
healers in the plant-food world, and luckily they are what gives our food so much flavor. While
you're on the journey to better health, start adding more spices to your dishes. Dessert is a great
place to start! Cinnamon, ginger, nutmeg and cardamom matched with dark chocolate are a perfect
team. Together they can not only activate your pleasure centers but they can also activate your
body's natural ability to heal itself. Healing through chocolate? Count me in!

THE GOODS

1 cup (240 g) smooth almond butter (see Bai's Tip)

2 tbsp (30 ml) melted coconut oil, plus 1 tsp solid coconut oil

¼ cup (60 ml) pure maple syrup

1 tsp ground cinnamon

¼ tsp ground nutmeg

¼ tsp ground cardamom

1 tsp pure vanilla extract

1 cup (96 g) almond flour (see Bai's Tip)

¼ tsp salt

1 cup (170 g) vegan dark chocolate chips

½ tsp ground ginger

THE METHOD

In a large bowl, mix together the almond butter, melted coconut oil, maple syrup, cinnamon, nutmeg, cardamom and vanilla. Mix in the flour and salt. It will seem like a lot at first, but the almond butter will soak up all the flour.

Grab a 9 x 9-inch (23 x 23–cm) baking pan and line it with parchment paper. Scoop the almond mixture into the prepared baking pan. Flatten the mixture with a spatula, so it's all even and smooth. Place the pan in the freezer while you melt the chocolate.

Melt the chocolate in a double boiler over low heat, stirring the chocolate constantly with your rubber spatula. When the chocolate is half melted, add the solid coconut oil and ginger. Once the chocolate has fully melted, remove it from the heat and grab your almond mixture from the freezer. Pour the chocolate over the top of the almond mixture and freeze them for 15 minutes. Once the chocolate has set, remove the almond mixture from the freezer and slice it into bars. Store the bars in the fridge and savor every bite.

BAI'S TIP: Allergic to almonds or nuts in general? Swap out the almond butter for sunflower seed butter and the almond flour for oat flour!

Makes 12 bars

NEW YORK–STYLE MATCHA CHEESECAKE

Some people say that cheesecake dates all the way back to AD 230, while New Yorkers claim that a cheesecake wasn't a cheesecake until it hit NYC. New York does have a way of putting its own take on things, and in honor of my father, this cheesecake has New York written all over it. Not only do you get those classic cheesecake vibes, but it's also plant-based and gluten-free. Unlike a typical cheesecake recipe with lots of eggs, dairy products and complicated instructions, this recipe is as simple as throwing everything into your blender and popping it in the oven! Matcha is the perfect addition to this recipe, as its subtle flavor adds a slight umami vibe while matching perfectly with the cinnamon and adding a gorgeous green color. This is an authentic, ridiculously good cheesecake that'll turn even the most old-school, stubborn New Yorkers into believers in the power of plants!

THE GOODS

CRUST

1 cup (180 g) raw almonds

½ cup (58 g) raw walnuts

6 pitted Medjool dates

½ tsp ground cinnamon

2 tbsp (20 g) coconut sugar

1 tbsp (15 ml) melted coconut oil

CHEESECAKE

1 cup (150 g) raw cashews, soaked in cool water overnight and drained

2 (8-oz [227-g]) containers plain vegan cream cheese

¼ cup (60 ml) coconut cream

2 tbsp (18 g) tapioca flour

¾ cup (180 ml) pure maple syrup

½ tsp pure vanilla extract

1 tbsp (15 ml) fresh lemon juice

1½ tsp (3 g) matcha powder

THE METHOD

Preheat the oven to 350°F (177°C). Line the bottom of a 9-inch (23-cm) springform pan or a 9 x 9–inch (23 x 23–cm) baking dish with parchment paper.

To make the crust, combine the almonds, walnuts, dates, cinnamon and sugar in a food processor. Process the ingredients until the mixture is homogenous. Process on high speed, and slowly pour the coconut oil through the top hole of the food processor. Process until the mixture begins to hold together.

Press the crust down evenly and tightly into the bottom of the prepared pan. Bake the crust for 5 minutes.

While the crust is baking, make the cheesecake. In a blender, combine the cashews, cream cheese, coconut cream, tapioca flour, maple syrup, vanilla and lemon juice. Blend the ingredients for about 30 seconds, or until the mixture is super smooth. Remove about ¼ cup (60 g) of the white cheesecake mixture from the blender and set it aside. Add the matcha to the blender, blend it into the remaining cheesecake mixture until it's smooth and then pour the green cheesecake filling into the crust. To create the swirl, use a swirling motion to drizzle the white cheesecake filling on the top of the green filling. Using a toothpick, swirl the white and the green together until you get a pattern you're happy with.

Bake the cheesecake for 25 minutes. You'll know it's done when it's no longer jiggly in the center and the filling has puffed up. Let the cheesecake cool completely, and then let it set in the fridge for 6 hours for the best results.

BAI'S TIP: If you want to switch it up, you can add 2 tablespoons (14 g) of cacao powder instead of matcha, or you can keep it classic with no flavoring!

Makes 1 (9-inch [23-cm]) cheesecake

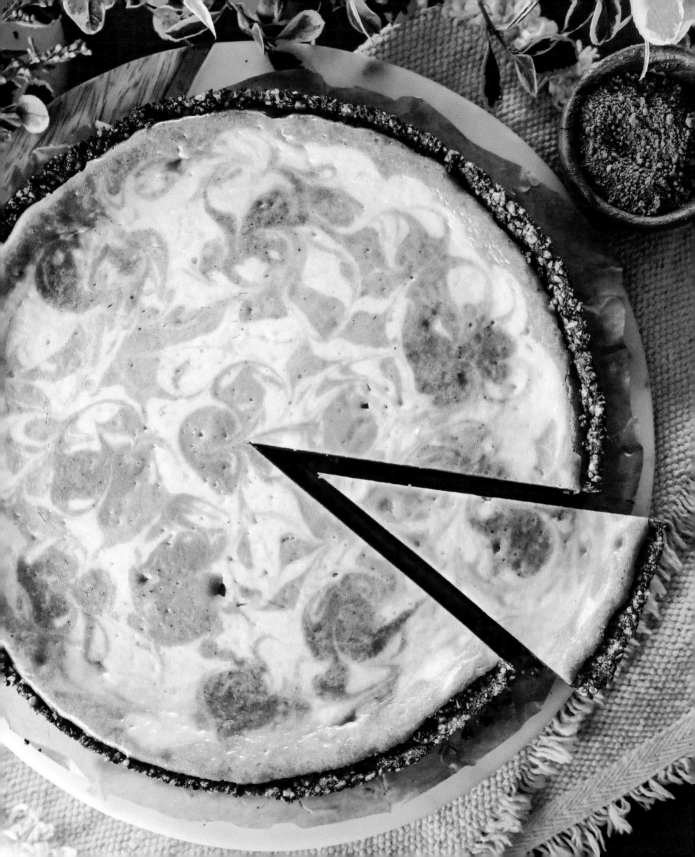

MOCHA CHOCOLATE CAKE WITH AVOCADO FROSTING

Nothing says bliss quite like baking a cake. There was a time when I worked for one of the top pastry chefs and bakers in San Francisco. During that time, I learned a few key things about baking cakes. The first is to relax into the process. It's not something to be rushed—even when you're doing it professionally, it's a process that's meant to be enjoyed fully. So put on music, get into your vibe and enjoy yourself! The second thing is to use creative ingredients to complete simple ideas and rich flavors. With coffee undertones, rich cacao and almond meal, this cake will become one of your new obsessions. I even use avocado to replace butter in my frosting. All of these elements make for an incredible cake that just happens to be gluten-free and vegan!

My final words of cake wisdom? Use a rubber spatula to get every last drop from your bowl into your cake pan! Every. Last. Drop! This is an epic cake for any occasion and will take care of cake fanatics, kiddos, most people with food allergies and—most importantly—you!

THE GOODS

CAKE

Coconut oil, for greasing

1 cup (112 g) cacao powder, sifted

1 cup (120 g) cassava flour, sifted

2¼ cups (216 g) almond flour

2 tsp (8 g) baking powder, sifted

1½ tsp (6 g) baking soda

1 tsp salt

¾ cup (120 g) coconut sugar

1 cup (260 g) unsweetened applesauce

1¼ cups (300 ml) plant milk

1 tsp pure vanilla extract

2 tbsp (30 ml) melted coconut oil

2 tbsp (30 g) smooth almond butter

¼ cup (60 ml) pure maple syrup

1 cup (240 ml) hot coffee

FROSTING

2 large avocados

¼ cup (28 g) cacao powder

¼ cup (60 ml) plus 1 tbsp (15 ml) pure maple syrup

½ (4-oz [113-g]) vegan dark chocolate bar, melted

½ tsp pure vanilla extract

1 cup (160 g) shaved dark chocolate

THE METHOD

First, preheat the oven to 350°F (177°C). Grease two 9-inch (23-cm) cake pans with coconut oil. Line the bottoms of the pans with parchment paper if you want the cakes to release more easily from the pans later on.

In a large bowl, sift together the cacao and cassava flour. Next, add the almond flour, baking powder, baking soda, salt and sugar. If any of the dry ingredients are clumpy, use the sifter or a whisk to break up any large clumps as you add them to the bowl.

In this order, add the applesauce, milk, vanilla, oil, almond butter and maple syrup. Using a whisk, stir the ingredients as you add them until they become a beautiful chocolate cake batter. Next, add the hot coffee slowly while stirring the batter. The batter will be thin, but don't worry, this is exactly what you want; don't overmix the batter.

Pour 3 cups (720 ml) of the batter into each of the prepared cake pans. Bake the cakes for 30 minutes, until a toothpick inserted into the center comes out clean.

As the cakes bake, make the frosting. In a food processor, combine the avocados, cacao, maple syrup, melted chocolate and vanilla. Process the ingredients until they are very smooth. You don't want any chunks. This will be the frosting for the cake, so be sure not to eat it all beforehand.

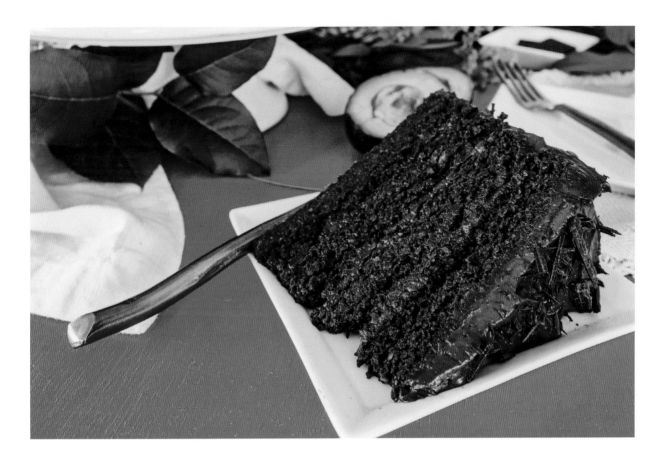

BAI'S TIPS: *Feel free to double the recipe and create a 4-layer cake!*

To make cupcakes, line a cupcake pan with parchment liners. Fill the muffin cavities almost to the top with the cake batter (this recipe doesn't rise very much), and bake the cupcakes for 35 to 40 minutes, until a toothpick inserted into the center of a cupcake comes out clean. Let the cupcakes cool completely, then top them with the frosting and shaved chocolate! Makes 16 cupcakes.

Once the cakes are done, pull them out of the oven and let them cool for 3 to 5 minutes. Using a butter knife, gently cut around the edges of the cake pans and remove each whole cake from its pan. Transfer the cakes to a cooling rack. Let them cool for 30 to 45 minutes, until they are almost fully cooled.

Place one of the cakes on a large serving plate. Using a spatula, create a ¼-inch (6-mm)-thick layer of chocolate frosting on the top of the cake. Try to make it even, then carefully top the frosting layer with the other cake. The trick is to set it down on top of the frosting without crushing it, in order to avoid squeezing frosting out of the cake's sides. Once both cakes are stacked, cover the entire cake with frosting. This is the fun part. Leave no spot untouched. Once fully frosted, sprinkle or gently press the chocolate shavings into the frosting. The frosted cake is ready to eat immediately!

Makes 1 (9-inch [23-cm]) double layer cake

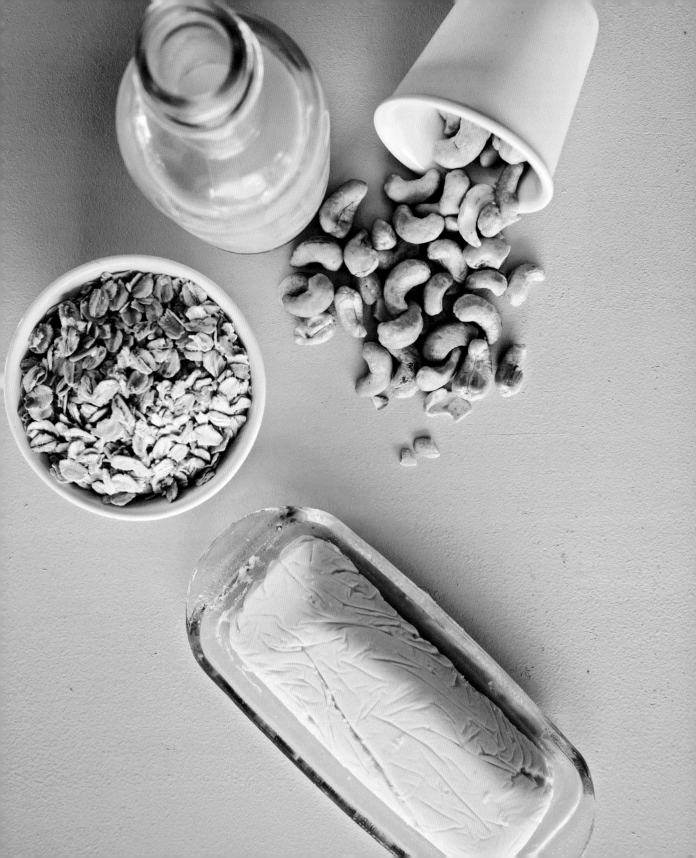

THE *Essentials*

This chapter is one of the most important concepts in this book, as the essentials will make or break your ability to be consistent not just with healthy eating but with a plant-based diet too. A guide to plant-based staples is something I wish I'd had when I was transitioning to a vegan diet.

Staples are important because they form the building blocks of our recipes, our calories and how we experience flavor. For example, common staples are condiments, dairy products, dips, snacks, broth and bread, just to name a few. Every single person has a completely different set of staples in their cabinets and refrigerator. Whenever I do a complete kitchen overhaul with a client, I learn a lot about how they eat, how they view food and what stage of their health journey they're in by looking at their staples. If you were to look at all the staples in your kitchen, what would they say about you and where you are in your health journey?

When you're looking to rethink your lifestyle, the essentials are where you should start. First, look at the nutrition labels of everything in your cabinets and your fridge. There are a few things to look out for when deciding if you'll keep or toss a certain item. Check the number of ingredients first. If it has a ridiculously long list of ingredients, you're looking at a highly processed food, which can be hard for your body to process and can be damaging to your health. For instance, something as simple as a carton of veggie broth can have upwards of 50 ingredients. Always look out for sneaky sugars, hydrogenated oils, food colorings and other food additives. Avoid high-fructose corn syrup, palm oil, canola oil, natural flavors, shortening, artificial sweeteners and sodium nitrate. Eliminating these things from your kitchen can be an overwhelming process at first, but the more you continue to educate yourself on the foods that go inside your body, the more control you'll have over your health.

Consuming cleaner essentials can be as simple as just switching the brand you buy or beginning to make your own to get on the right track. There are many staples that you can buy at the grocery store; however, the best bet is to make your own at home! The ones I make all the time are quite easy to put together, call for inexpensive ingredients, are much more flavorful and are healthier than anything you can buy at the store. This way, you know exactly what's going inside.

You can reduce food waste and boost your immune system by making your own veggie broth (page 170). Avoid preservatives and excessive sugar by making your own plant milk and yogurt (page 162 and page 169). Level-up your meals with things like my Herbed Creamy Feta (page 166), Cashew Cream (page 173) and Seeded Herbed Spelt Bread (page 178). Get ready for a major upgrade as you cook your way through this chapter. These essentials are the building blocks of plant-based cooking, and by mastering these concepts, you are that much closer to truly thriving from the inside out!

NOT YOUR MAMA'S SALTED BUTTER

There's nothing quite like the essence of butter. This staple has a long history across the globe. As a French-trained chef and person of Eastern European descent, I saw butter in practically everything in my culinary schoolbooks and in my family's recipes when I was growing up. Butter is a simple way to add an incredible amount of flavor and fat to almost any dish at any step in the cooking process. Sure, you could go buy margarine or vegan butter alternatives, but are they really that much better for you? With all those hydrogenated oils and preservatives, none of those have lived up to the hype of real butter—until now. With this simple and delicious buttery recipe, you avoid the harmful effects of dairy, hydrogenated oils, preservatives and excessive sodium. All you need is a blender and some patience while the butter sets. The result is all you really wanted in the first place: incredible flavor and the versatility to be used in any recipe requiring butter. This'll make you go, "Mmmmm." Every. Single. Time.

THE GOODS

¼ cup (38 g) raw cashews, soaked in cool water overnight or in hot water for 15 minutes and drained

½ tsp apple cider vinegar

1 cup (240 ml) refined melted coconut oil (see Bai's Tips)

½ cup (120 ml) unsweetened oat milk

1 tsp salt

THE METHOD

In a high-powered blender, combine the cashews, vinegar, oil, milk and salt. Blend the ingredients for about 60 seconds, until the butter mixture is smooth.

Line an 8 x 8–inch (20 x 20–cm) glass baking dish or a butter mold that can hold 2 cups (480 ml) with parchment paper or plastic wrap. Pour the butter mixture into your prepared container. Cover the container, transfer it to the fridge and allow the butter to chill for at least 4 hours, preferably up to overnight. This butter will last in the fridge for 9 to 12 days, and you can freeze half of the batch if you need to.

BAI'S TIPS: Make sure to get refined coconut oil for this recipe, so that you'll avoid the intense coconut taste of unrefined coconut oil!

When sautéing veggies with this butter, make sure to do so over low heat, as the oil has a very low smoking point. For high-heat sautéing, I prefer avocado oil or veggie broth.

Makes 1½ cups (360 g)

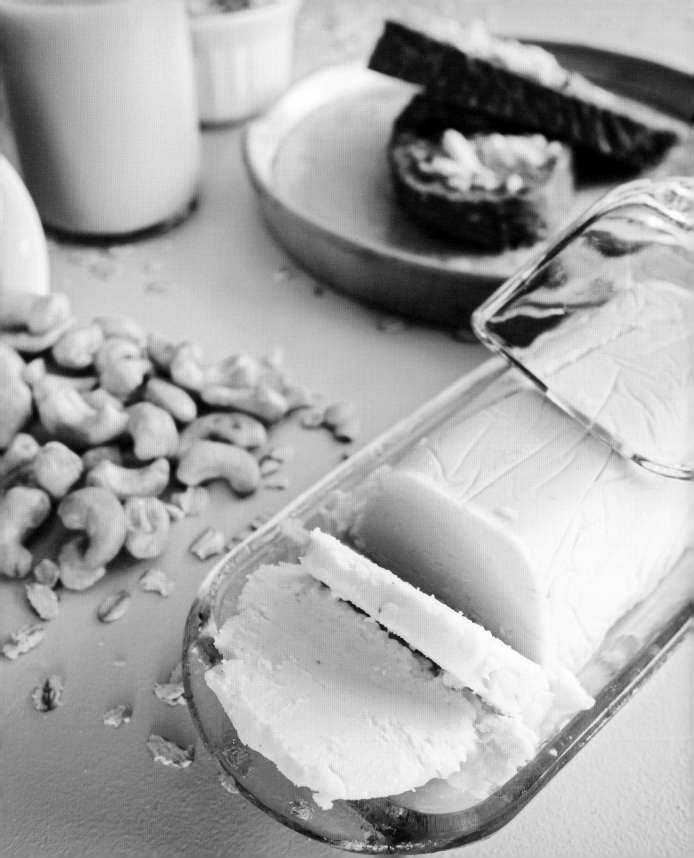

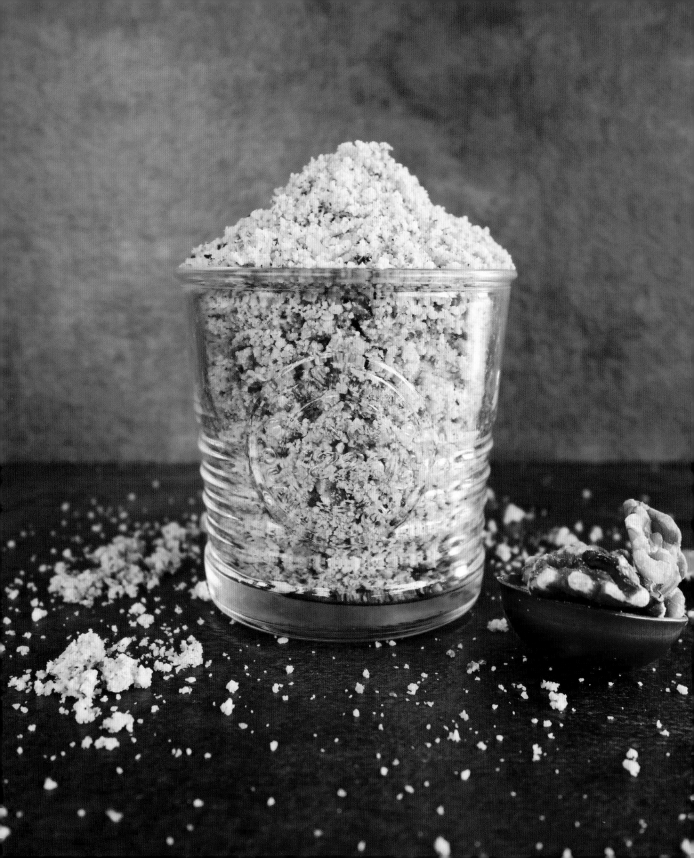

WALNUT PARM

Craving a cheesy, salty topping to your favorite meal? Not only will this nut-based Parm satisfy all of those cravings, but you can make it in under five minutes. This recipe reminds me of the processed Parm in the green shaker that we '90s kids would dump over everything we could. This recipe gives you that perfect pizza topping without any of the additives, hormones, preservatives or BS! This isn't shreddy, melty Parm, but it still goes perfectly with a tray of lasagna or a big ol' bowl of pasta. The winning touch? Walnuts are a prebiotic, meaning that these little guys are a dream for your gut's microbiome. Happy tummy, happy cravings, happy kids, happy you!

THE GOODS

1 cup (115 g) raw walnuts
¼ cup (30 g) hemp seeds
1 tsp nutritional yeast
1 tsp garlic powder
1 tsp salt

THE METHOD

In a dry blender, combine the walnuts, hemp seeds, nutritional yeast, garlic powder and salt. A dry blender is key, so that you can avoid any clumps! Blend the ingredients on low speed for 5 seconds, then blend on high speed for 2 to 3 seconds, until you get a powdery texture similar to almond meal.

Store the Parm in a medium Mason jar or other airtight container for up to 2 weeks. If you live in a warm, sunny climate like I do, you may want to store it in the refrigerator to keep the integrity of the seasoning.

BAI'S TIP: When you are traveling, keep a little jar of this Parm in your bag to spice up any boring airport meal!

Makes 1¼ cups (155 g)

CASHEW-HEMP MILK

Many years ago, I was incredibly skeptical about nut milks, as I believe we all have been at some point. Slowly and surely over the past decade, nut milks started popping up everywhere. Nowadays, there are just as many plant milk varieties on the shelves as dairy options. So why make your own? Besides avoiding dairy production—which can be so harmful to animals, the environment and our bodies—when you start to get in a groove of making and drinking your own plant milk on a regular basis, you also avoid all of the fillers, gums, preservatives, added sugars and other BS that can be found in some store-bought plant milks. But even beyond all of that: Are you ready for the best milk you've ever had in your life? This specific blend of ingredients is the bee's knees! I've seen this milk recipe alone change the way people think of plant-based food. It's fatty from the cashews, thickened and slightly sweetened from the dates and full of plant protein. No nut-milk bag is required—all you need is a standard mesh strainer. Plus it uses easy-to-find ingredients. This is it. The one you've been waiting for.

THE GOODS

1 cup (150 g) raw cashews (see Bai's Tips)

2 tbsp (16 g) hemp seeds

1 cup (240 ml) hot water

6 medium pitted Medjool dates (see Bai's Tips)

¼ tsp salt

6 cups (1.4 L) filtered water

THE METHOD

In a medium bowl, combine the cashews and hemp seeds. Pour the hot water over them and let them soak for 15 minutes. This step is important, as it allows the cashews to get nice and creamy. It's also very helpful for digestion—a win-win!

Drain the cashews and hemp seeds in a fine-mesh strainer. Transfer the cashews and hemp seeds to a blender. Add the dates, salt and filtered water. Blend the ingredients on high speed for 1 minute. The mixture will start to get white and foamy at the top. Strain the mixture through a mesh strainer into a 2-quart (2-L) Mason jar, secure the jar's lid and transfer the milk to the fridge. This milk is incredibly delicious served cold, so make sure you chill it for a few hours before diving in!

Serve it with cereal or a Dark Chocolate Oatmeal Cookie Skillet (page 140). Or use it in your favorite recipes as a one-to-one milk substitute.

Store the milk in an airtight jar in the fridge for 1 week.

BAI'S TIPS: Use oats as a substitute for the cashews if needed.

If you're looking for a slightly sweeter milk, add 2 more pitted dates and ½ teaspoon of ground cinnamon.

You can easily cut the recipe in half for a single portion for the week. If you're looking to double the recipe, you'll need to make the milk in two batches, as it won't all fit in the blender!

Makes 2 quarts (2 L)

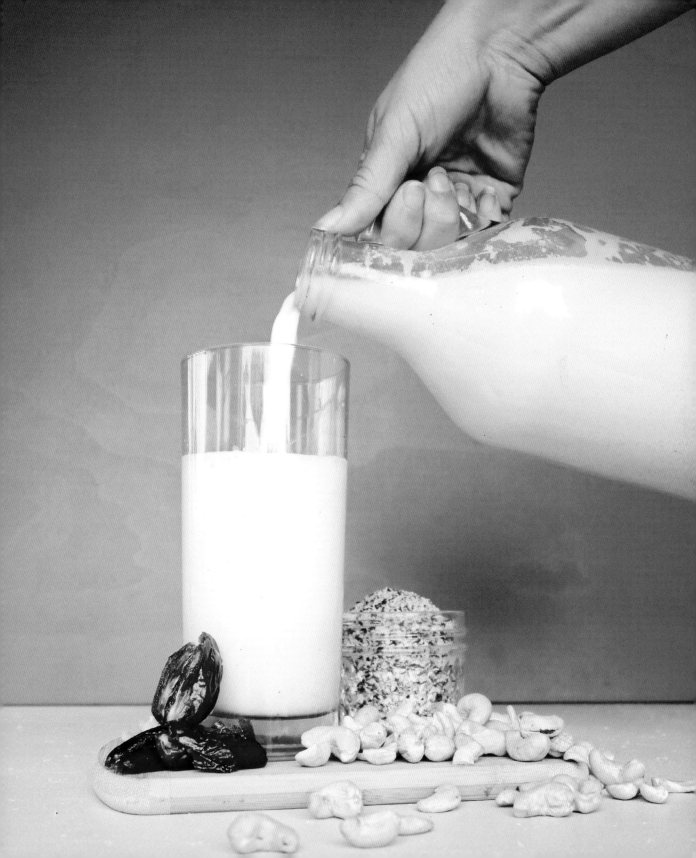

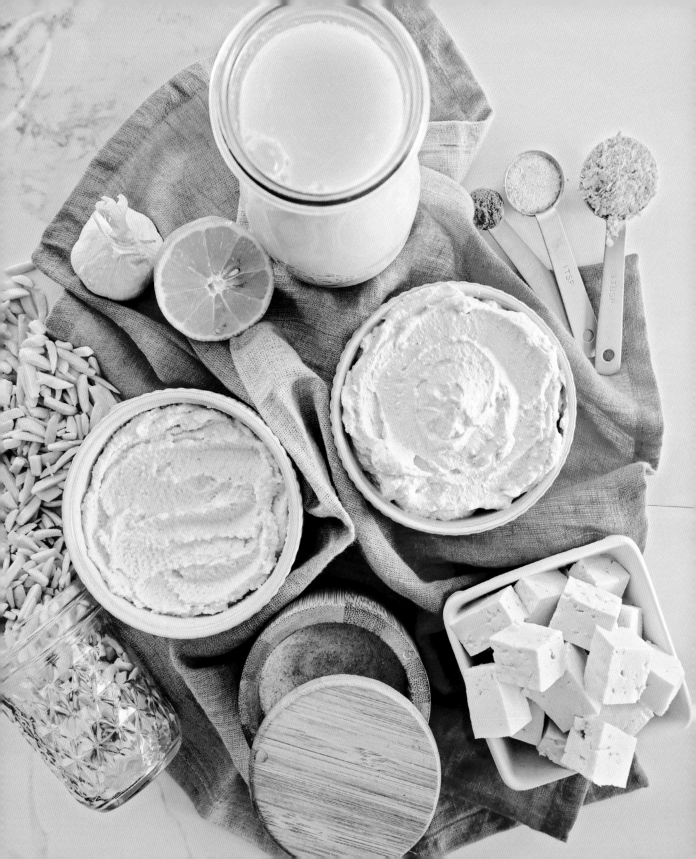

RICOTTA TWO WAYS

Creamy ricotta is a cooking staple and not something you should miss out on just because you're diving into the world of plant-based food. There are vegan ricottas you can buy at the store, but depending on where you live that may not be an option for you. Both of these recipes have simple ingredients that are easy to find and can work for most people. If you have a soy allergy, the almond ricotta is perfect for you. If you're allergic to nuts, the tofu ricotta has your name on it. Either way, both are creamy and delicious in classic recipes like lasagna (page 19). Try both of them in some of your favorite recipes—you'll be shocked at how you don't miss the animal-based version.

THE GOODS

ALMOND RICOTTA

1½ cups (159 g) whole or slivered blanched almonds

2 tbsp (30 ml) fresh lemon juice

1 tsp salt

3 cloves garlic, peeled

½ cup (120 ml) Cashew-Hemp Milk (page 162) or plant milk of choice, plus more as needed

TOFU RICOTTA

1 (14-oz [397-g]) block firm tofu, drained

1¼ tsp (6 g) salt

¼ tsp ground nutmeg

2 tbsp (10 g) nutritional yeast

2 tbsp (30 ml) fresh lemon juice

1 tsp garlic powder (optional)

THE METHOD

To make the almond ricotta, combine the almonds, lemon juice, salt, garlic and milk in a high-powered blender or food processor. Blend the ingredients on medium speed until they reach a smooth consistency. If your blender has a hard time making this ricotta smooth, you may need to add a few teaspoons (5 to 10 ml) of additional milk to smooth it out.

To make the tofu ricotta, combine the tofu, salt, nutmeg, nutritional yeast, lemon juice and garlic powder (if using) in a blender or food processor. Pulse the ingredients until they have a smooth and fluffy consistency.

Store the ricotta, covered, in your fridge for 7 to 8 days.

Makes 2 cups (310 g) almond ricotta and 1½ cups (410 g) tofu ricotta

HERBED CREAMY FETA

Are you ready for the amazing process of vegan cheesemaking? Although I will admit that it's intimidating at first, it truly is the best way to enjoy cheese while exploring the plant world. For me, cheese was one of the hardest things to give up while I was switching to a plant-based diet, as a lot of the processed vegan cheeses out there just don't compare to the real thing. I made it my mission to create delectable and crave-worthy cheeses that will have you coming back for more! This feta cheese, with a flavor reminiscent of goat cheese, is a hybrid of cheeses made out of plants. The ingredients are easy to find, inexpensive, high in protein and nut allergy–friendly. Add this feta to your favorite Greek salads, sandwiches, tofu scrambles, summer cheese boards and more. You will need some patience to let this cheese solidify, but trust me when I say that it's worth the wait!

THE GOODS

1 (14-oz [397-g]) block firm tofu, drained

2 tbsp (40 g) miso paste

3 tbsp (45 ml) lemon juice

1 tbsp (15 ml) white wine vinegar

½ cup (120 ml) melted refined coconut oil (see Bai's Tips on page 158)

2 tsp (10 g) salt

1 tsp finely chopped fresh rosemary

1 tsp finely chopped fresh thyme

1 tsp finely chopped fresh sage

THE METHOD

Pat the tofu dry with a clean kitchen towel, then wrap it in the towel. Press the tofu for 15 minutes while it's wrapped in the towel: You can use your hands to press it lightly, but I like to put it under a carton of veggie broth to press out more of the water.

Crumble your block of tofu into a blender or food processor. Add the miso, lemon juice, vinegar, oil and salt. Blend the ingredients until they are smooth and creamy. Next, add the rosemary, thyme and sage and pulse the blender a few times until the herbs are well combined in the feta mixture.

Line a medium glass container with cheesecloth or plastic wrap, making sure to leave overhang to act as handles later. Transfer the feta mixture to the prepared container, smooth the top of the feta and cover the container with its lid. Refrigerate the feta for 6 to 8 hours.

Pull the block of feta out of the container using the overhanging cheesecloth and remove the cheesecloth. Store the feta for up to 1 week. I like to keep cut pieces in a glass jar with herbs and olive oil. So pretty for cheese boards!

Makes 1 (18-oz [510-g]) block

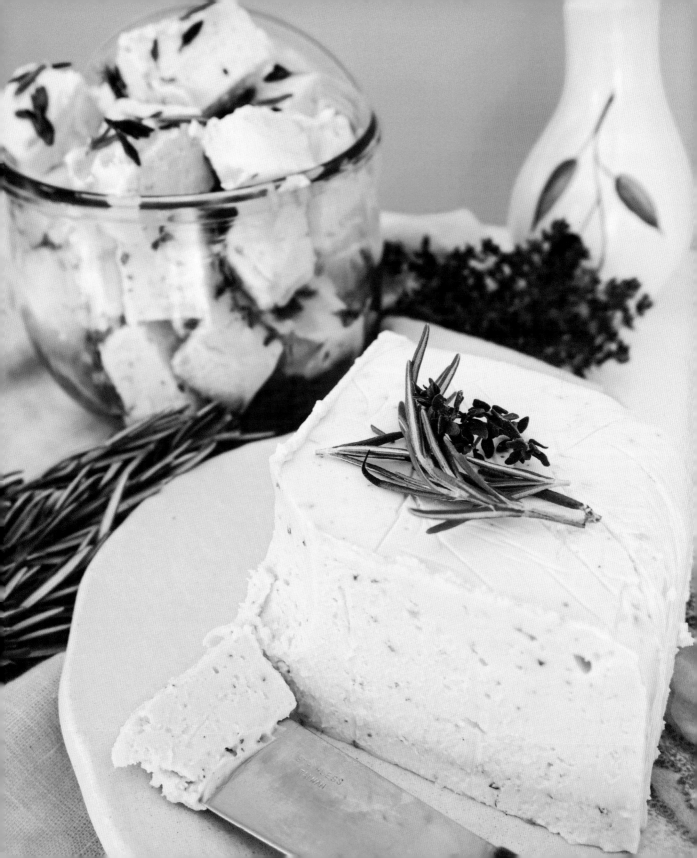

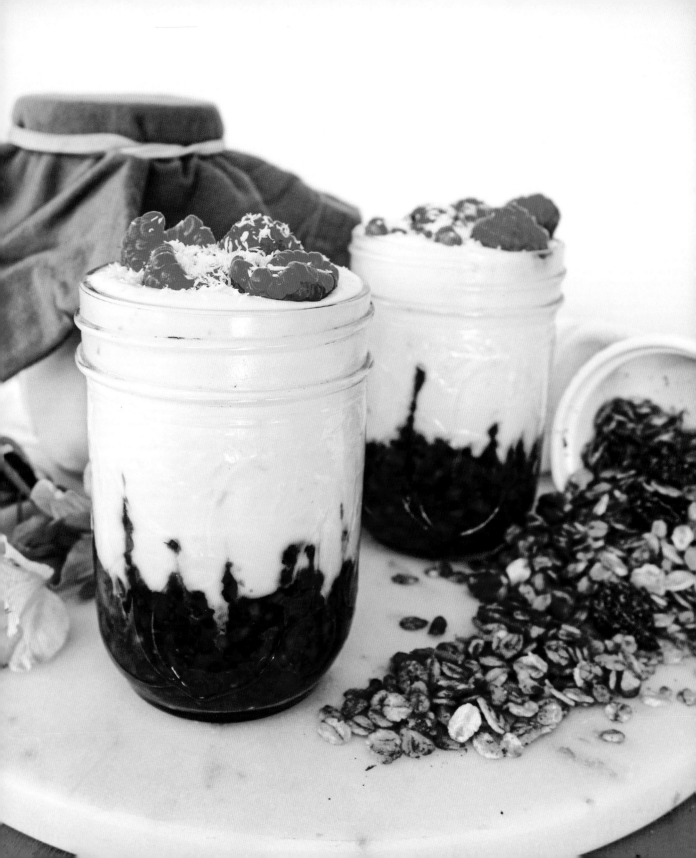

SLIGHTLY SWEET COCONUT YOGURT

Learning how to make your own yogurt will give you a new type of confidence in the kitchen. The plant-based yogurt at the store is getting better, but it's expensive and can be hard to find depending on where you live. Since accessibility, nutrition and flavor are some of our keys to success on a plant-based diet, access shouldn't stop at things we eat all the time like yogurt. The process to make yogurt is actually quite simple, but there are a few keys to help make you successful. The first is to find canned organic full-fat coconut milk that doesn't have added sugars or coconut water. This will give you a consistent flavor and texture. The second is to buy simple probiotic capsules that don't have prebiotics or any other vitamins in them—you can usually find them refrigerated in the supplements aisle. Finally, make sure you let the yogurt ferment in a cool spot on your counter that's not in direct sunlight. If you're making this midsummer without any AC, pop it into your cabinet—in a spot where you'll see it often—and it should be fine!

This yogurt is slightly sweetened to get the perfect yogurt flavor without all that added sugar. There is nothing better than fresh, house-fermented yogurt that you can make again whenever you run out! Serve it in smoothies, or with granola, or skip the sweetener and use it in savory recipes like Gluten-Free Garlic Naan (page 41). The possibilities are endless!

THE GOODS

1 (15-oz [443-ml]) can organic full-fat coconut milk

2 tbsp (18 g) tapioca flour

1 tbsp (15 ml) pure maple syrup (see Bai's Tip)

2 vegan probiotic capsules

THE METHOD

Sanitize a 16-ounce (454-g) Mason jar and a small saucepan with very hot water and soap. This will help get rid of any bacteria in the jar and saucepan, in order to get you the same results every time.

Place the milk in the saucepan. Heat the milk over low heat and whisk in your tapioca flour and maple syrup. Whisk the mixture for 2 to 4 minutes, until the milk starts to thicken and get hot. Remove the mixture from the heat and let it cool to room temperature, about 20 minutes.

After the mixture has cooled, open your probiotic capsules over the mixture and whisk their contents into the mixture thoroughly. Transfer the yogurt to your sanitized jar, top it with a clean cloth or terry towel and wrap a rubber band around the top to hold the cloth in place. Let the yogurt ferment on the counter for 24 to 48 hours. The longer it sits, the tangier it'll get, so it's up to you! You can taste it after 24 hours to see how it's progressing. I personally like my yogurt fermented for about 30 hours.

Once the yogurt is fully fermented to your liking, remove the cloth and replace it with a proper lid. Store the yogurt in your fridge for up to 1 week. I love it with Berrylicious Chia Jam (page 177), fruit and granola!

BAI'S TIP: *If you're making a dish that calls for unsweetened coconut yogurt, simply omit the maple syrup from this recipe.*

Makes 16 oz (473 mL)

IMMUNE-BOOSTING VEGGIE BROTH

Making your own veggie broth is a great way to reduce waste and save some money in the process. When I cook, I save all my onion and garlic skins, carrot tops, mushroom stems, broccoli stalks, fennel tops and the like to make a broth that costs nothing and limits the amount of food scraps getting thrown in the trash. Plus, homemade veggie broth is amazing for your gut health and can have just as many nutritional properties as bone broth. By making your own veggie broth, you support your gut, boost your immune system, save money, reduce food waste and give a helping hand to our environment. It's awesome how something so simple can be so impactful. This recipe is a great starting point—don't be afraid to mix it up with what you have on hand and add your scraps to this recipe!

THE GOODS

3 medium carrots, finely chopped

1 large leek, thickly sliced

Top from 1 medium fennel bulb, coarsely chopped (see Bai's Tips)

3 medium ribs celery, finely chopped

1 medium head garlic, cloves smashed, skins reserved

1 medium onion, sliced, skins reserved

3 tbsp (6 g) dried herbs of choice

8 cups (1.9 L) water

THE METHOD

In a large slow cooker, combine the carrots, leek, fennel tops, celery, garlic and garlic skins, onion and onion skins, herbs and water. Put the lid on the slow cooker and cook the broth on low for 12 to 24 hours. Strain the broth through a strainer over a large bowl. If you don't have a slow cooker, you can cook the broth in a large pot over low heat for 4 to 6 hours.

Pour or ladle the broth into a 2-quart (2-L) Mason jar or multiple smaller jars. Let the broth cool completely before putting a lid on the jar and storing it in the fridge. Use the broth within 10 days.

BAI'S TIPS: If 2 quarts (2 L) is way more than you'll use, just pour the broth into smaller freezer-safe Mason jars, leaving at least 2 inches (5 cm) of room on the top. Freeze the broth and use it whenever you need it!

Remember that your broth will take on whatever flavor you give it, so avoid jalapeño seeds unless you love spicy broths, and avoid veggies like cabbage, cauliflower and Brussels sprouts in excess.

You can use the bottom of the fennel bulb in the broth or save it for the Moroccan Lentil Soup (page 137) to utilize the broth and leftover fennel in one recipe!

Makes 2 quarts (2 L)

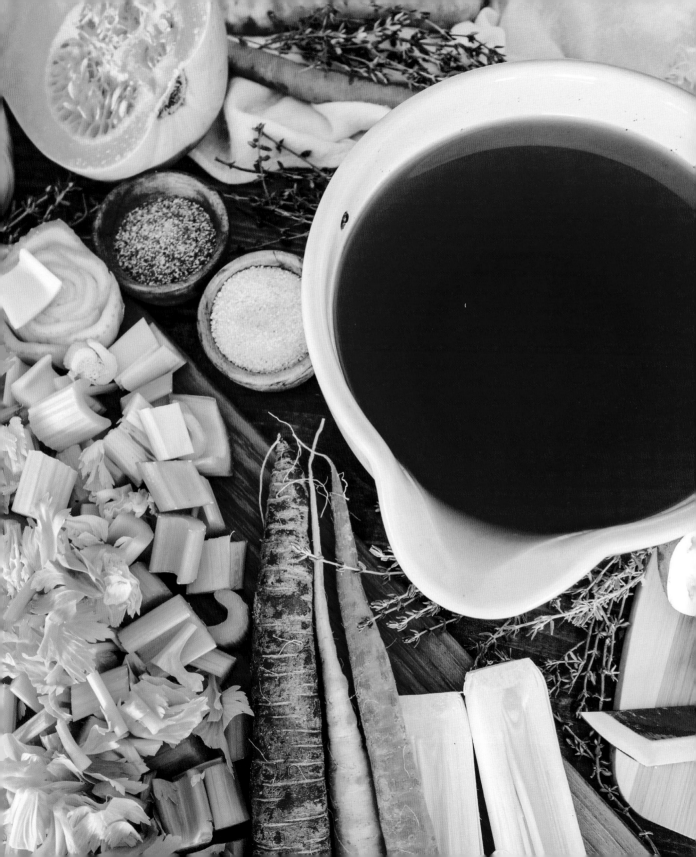

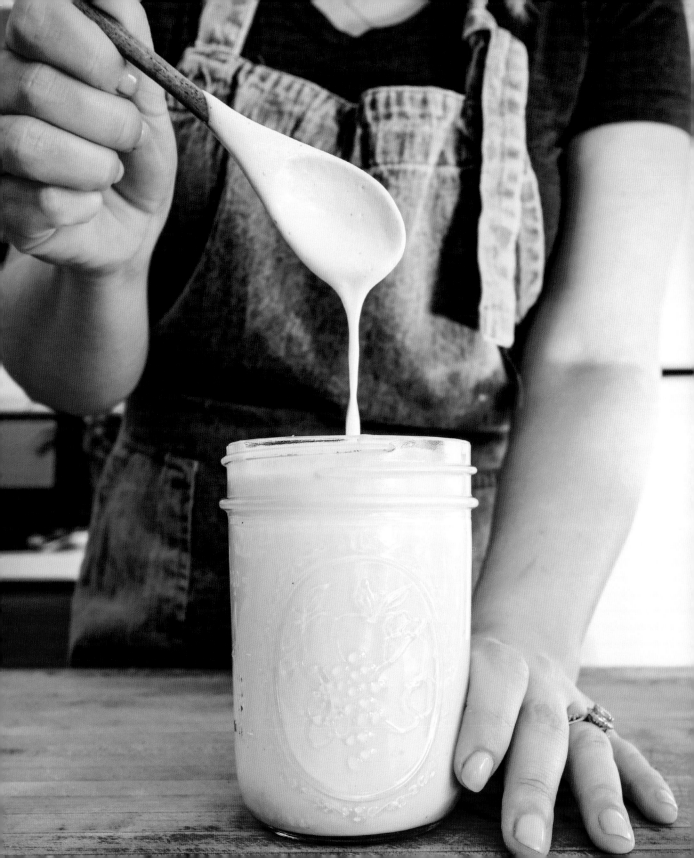

CASHEW CREAM

If I had to choose one plant-based staple to always have on hand, this would be it! Cashew cream can make your life in the kitchen incredibly easy and delicious. In fact, when you're first transitioning to a plant-based diet, cashew cream can make life a lot easier. It's the perfect replacement for sour cream, mayo and heavy cream in nonvegan recipes. I love it by itself on tacos, in soups and in tofu scrambles. You can also use it as a base for sauces, like a spicy aioli or a cilantro crema to add some excitement to your routine! Cashews are also known as nature's antidepressant and can literally make you happy when you eat them in moderation. Flavor, happy vibes and protein in a kitchen staple? Oh, yeah!

THE GOODS

2 cups (300 g) raw cashews, soaked in cool water overnight or in hot water for 15 minutes and drained

2 tsp (10 ml) white wine vinegar

2 tbsp (30 ml) fresh lemon juice

1 tsp salt

1¼ cups (300 ml) filtered water

THE METHOD

In a high-powered blender, combine the cashews, vinegar, lemon juice, salt and water. Blend the ingredients for 2 minutes, until they reach a very smooth and creamy texture.

Use the cashew cream immediately in a recipe or store it in the fridge for 7 to 8 days.

BAI'S TIP: Store this cream in a squeeze bottle in the fridge, so you can easily drizzle it over everything!

Makes 2 cups (480 ml)

PESTO ALMOND HUMMUS

It's important to give credit where credit is due: This recipe is all thanks to my husband, Steve. He's the dip and cheese master, and I owe this one to him. This is the perfect addition to any party platter or the ideal dip for a snack. This dip is a fun twist on traditional hummus and damn, it's ridiculously good and fluffy. The fat in the almonds gives this a flavor like no other. No soaking necessary on these nuts, as the blender breaks them up perfectly. Make this for your friends or keep it all for yourself. Either way, your next snack attack or party just got a major upgrade.

THE GOODS

1½ cups (270 g) raw almonds

1 tbsp (15 ml) olive oil

½ tsp salt

3 tbsp (45 ml) fresh lemon juice

1 tsp liquid aminos

3 cloves garlic, peeled

1 packed cup (120 g) fresh basil
(see Bai's Tip)

1¾ cups (420 ml) water

THE METHOD

In a high-powered blender or food processor, combine the almonds, oil, salt, lemon juice, liquid aminos, garlic, basil and water. Blend the ingredients for 2 minutes, until they reach a smooth consistency.

Transfer the hummus to a serving dish and serve it with toast points or chopped veggies.

BAI'S TIP: Replace the basil with 1 teaspoon of chipotle powder and 1 teaspoon of ground cumin to change it from a pesto to a spicy Southwest hummus!

Makes 3 cups (720 g)

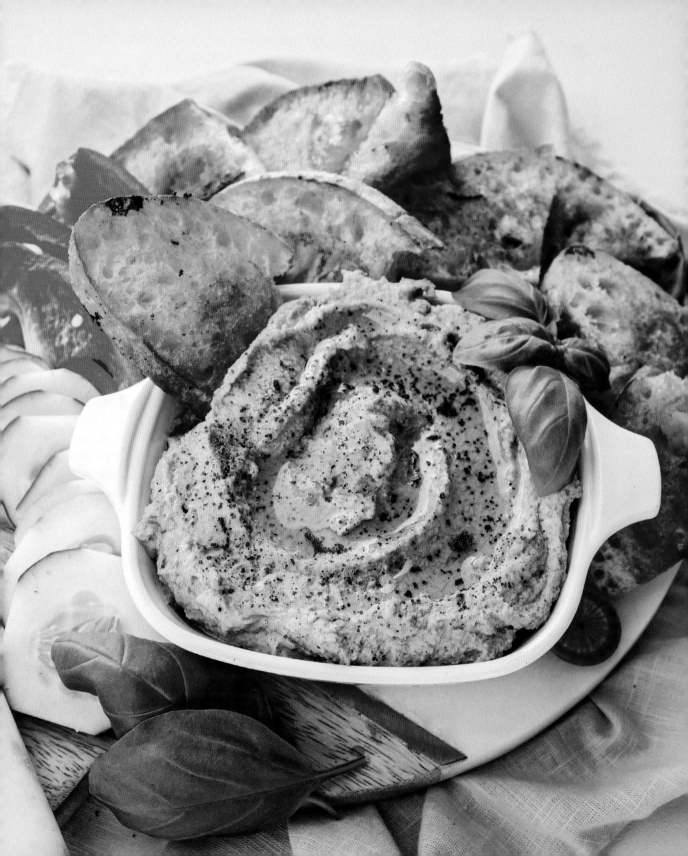

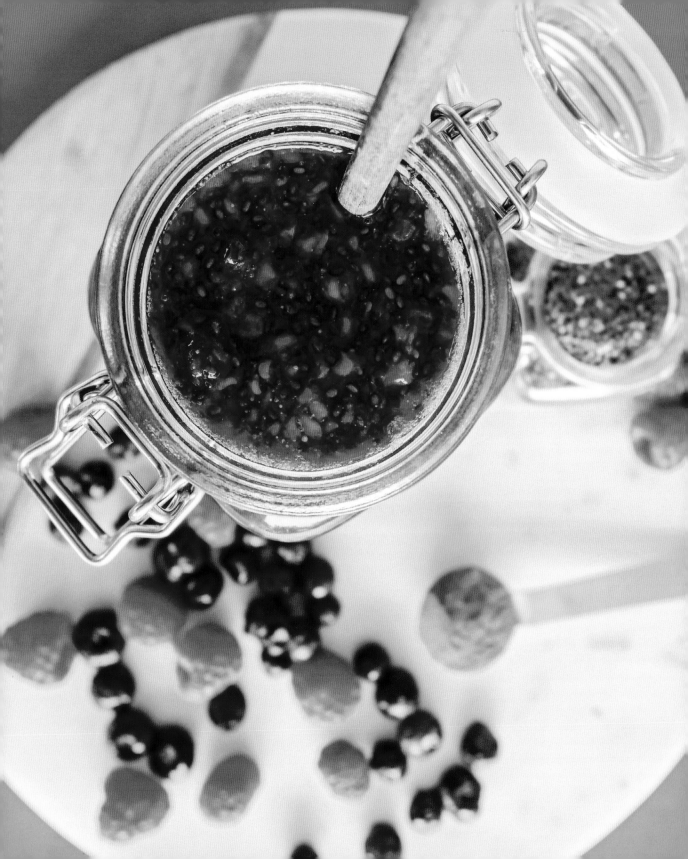

BERRYLICIOUS CHIA JAM

Who doesn't love a good jam? Jam reminds me of those little personal-sized containers of jam you would get when you were at your favorite breakfast spot with Grandma. Jam is an old-school way to preserve fruit and add a little sweetness to many different things. The problem with traditional jam or jelly is that it's filled with refined sugar and gelatin. Eating something incredibly sugary first thing in the morning can spike your blood sugar and isn't the most ideal way to get your day started. Gelatin is made from animal by-products—without totally grossing you out, let's just say there's a better way to get that jammy texture we're lookin' for. Chia seeds are an incredible source of protein, with 5 grams in just 1 ounce (28 g), and they are super absorbent and gelatinous. Berries are high in antioxidants and flavor and very low in sugar. The best part to all of this? This recipe takes only ten minutes to cook, and you can swap out the recommended berries for whatever is in season for you at the time. Use this jam to top your pancakes, toast and oats. Say hello to delicious, healthy and fruity breakfast vibes!

THE GOODS

1½ cups (200 g) fresh or frozen raspberries

1½ cups (200 g) fresh or frozen blueberries

1 cup (240 ml) water

½ tsp ground cinnamon

1 tbsp (15 ml) pure date or maple syrup

3 tbsp (30 g) chia seeds

THE METHOD

In a large sauté pan over medium heat, combine the raspberries, blueberries and water. Stir in the cinnamon and date syrup. Cook the mixture for 5 minutes, stirring it occasionally while smashing the fruit.

Add the chia seeds and stir to incorporate them evenly throughout the mixture. Cook the mixture for 5 minutes, stirring it every minute or so, then remove it from the heat. Let the jam sit for 10 minutes to cool, and let that smell of cinnamon and cooked fruit fill your kitchen with so much goodness!

Store the jam in a medium jar in your fridge for up to 10 days.

Makes 2 cups (640 g)

SEEDED HERBED SPELT BREAD

Regardless of whether you've never attempted to make your own bread before or if you're a seasoned pro, this bread recipe will easily win your heart. This recipe is made with alkalizing spelt flour. Spelt in itself is a super grain, and it's so flavorful! It's packed with essential nutrients and it's good for your heart and gut. Additionally, this recipe involves a fermentation process, so although you'll have to wait a bit, the fermentation contributes to the incredible flavor of this bread and helps with digestion. This bread will rock your world, your taste buds and your body.

THE GOODS

3½ cups (560 g) spelt flour, divided

2½ tsp (8 g) active dry yeast

1½ tsp (8 g) table or Himalayan pink salt

1 tbsp (3 g) dried or finely chopped fresh thyme

1 tbsp (3 g) dried or finely chopped fresh basil

1 tbsp (3 g) dried or finely chopped fresh rosemary

1 tbsp (8 g) poppy seeds, divided

2 tbsp (18 g) sesame seeds, divided

2 tbsp (20 g) coconut sugar

1¾ cups (420 ml) room-temperature filtered water

1 tsp flaky sea salt

1 tsp granulated garlic

BAI'S TIP: To make this into a round loaf, place a 5-quart (5-L) Dutch oven in your oven when you preheat it. Line the Dutch oven with parchment paper and place the dough inside. Top the dough with the seed mixture, make a few slices on the top, cover and bake the bread for 30 minutes. Uncover the Dutch oven and bake the bread for 15 more minutes. Remove the bread to a rack to cool.

THE METHOD

In a large bowl, combine 3 cups (480 g) of the spelt flour, yeast, Himalayan pink salt, thyme, basil, rosemary, ½ tablespoon (4 g) of the poppy seeds, 1 tablespoon (9 g) of the sesame seeds and the sugar. Mix the ingredients with a fork until everything is well combined. Slowly add the water and mix the dough with a fork until the water has been absorbed. Don't overmix this dough or attempt to form it into a ball. It will be wet and messy, and that's exactly what you want. Cover the bowl loosely with a lid; make sure it's not completely airtight. Let the dough sit on the counter to ferment and rise for at least 6 hours and no more than 24 hours. The dough will double in size. The more you let it ferment, the stronger sourdough taste you'll get.

Preheat your oven to 450°F (232°C). Line a 5 x 9–inch (13 x 23–cm) loaf pan with parchment paper. In a small bowl, mix together the remaining ½ tablespoon (4 g) of poppy seeds, 1 tablespoon (9 g) of sesame seeds, flaky sea salt and granulated garlic. Set this mixture aside.

Grab your bowl with the dough and remove the lid. Sprinkle 2 to 3 tablespoons (20 to 30 g) of the remaining flour over the top of the dough. Start to release it from the sides of the bowl with your hands, but keep it in the bowl. Knead the dough in the bowl five or six times, dusting it with a bit of the remaining flour as needed. The dough will still be a little flimsy and tacky to the touch.

Release the dough into the lined loaf pan and cover the top of the dough with your seed mixture. Make a few shallow diagonal slices on the top. Let the dough rest for 10 minutes, and then bake it for 35 minutes. It will puff up and be nice and golden brown on top when it's done. Remove the bread from the oven and use the parchment paper to immediately remove it from the loaf pan. Let the bread cool on a rack for about 30 minutes before serving it. Yum!

Keep the bread in an airtight bag on the counter for 4 days, and then move it to the fridge. If you want to make this bread in big batches to freeze, slice it first and put it into an airtight container before freezing it.

Makes 1 loaf

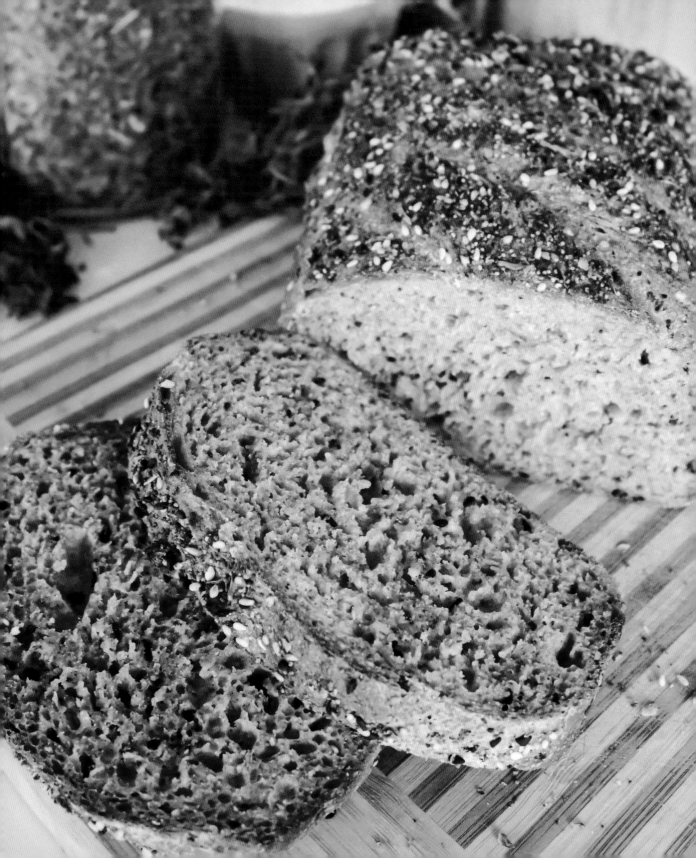

MAKING A *Solid Plan*

So you've cooked or flipped your way here, and you could be thinking, "Okay . . . now what?" This right here is the work, the daily life in the midst of chaos. How you show up for yourself on a weekly basis will determine how consistent you can be with your health and your ability to make change in this world by what you eat. The number one stumbling block I see with people starting a plant-based diet or a healthier eating routine is that they have great ideas and great intentions but no follow-through. The reason this happens is that they don't have the right plan. We can put intentions toward something all we want, but if we don't make a plan with actionable steps, it's just another idea that gets lost in the universe.

This is true with anything in life and is especially true with creating new habits around cooking and food. So, many times you'll get motivated and juiced to be on track that week: You will hit the grocery store, buy a ton of produce, and toss it in the fridge, and before you know it, it's nine days later and all that kale you bought is slimy and hard to even look at, let alone eat!

The simple remedy to this problem is making a solid plan and actually sticking to it! Use the recipes in this book to plan out at least some of your meals for the week. Even planning out a sauce, a salad, a few staples and a smoothie or two can be a help during the week. Bonus points if you actually get around to meal-prepping any of it!

I don't fully believe in the idea of meal-prepping every meal and eating the same meal for the whole week. I do believe in making your lunches, prepping your staples and planning your breakfasts and dinners. If you can take some time to partially prep your dinners, then you're setting yourself up for success. For example, I love to prep my Curry Paste (page 45), Immune-Boosting Veggie Broth (page 170), Cashew-Hemp Milk (page 162) and the Rustic Italian Chopped Salad (page 130) on Sundays. Doing so gives me a boost for a night of dinner, sets me up for a soup to make later in the week, refills my milk carton and gets lunch ready. You can do all of that in fewer than 90 minutes too!

Over the next few pages you'll find three of my favorite meal plans that have similar ingredients, are easy to create together while multitasking and create a delicious meal all together. I hope this can inspire you to create your own version for what's in season, what you're in the mood for and what will work best with your schedule. When you're making your plan, think about how much time you have to prep, how much you'll be working out that week, if you'll be eating out and how intense your work schedule will be. Write it all down, and with that info, make a plan for food. Decide how much you want to cook and what you're willing to go out for! Remember, put your own oxygen mask on first, so that you can then be your best self for your family, your work and your life.

This style of planning will set you up to succeed beyond the pages of this book. It'll help you feel organized and it will be the difference of your making a few recipes versus really thriving in this lifestyle. Let these three meal guides steer you in the right direction and you take it from there. You got this!

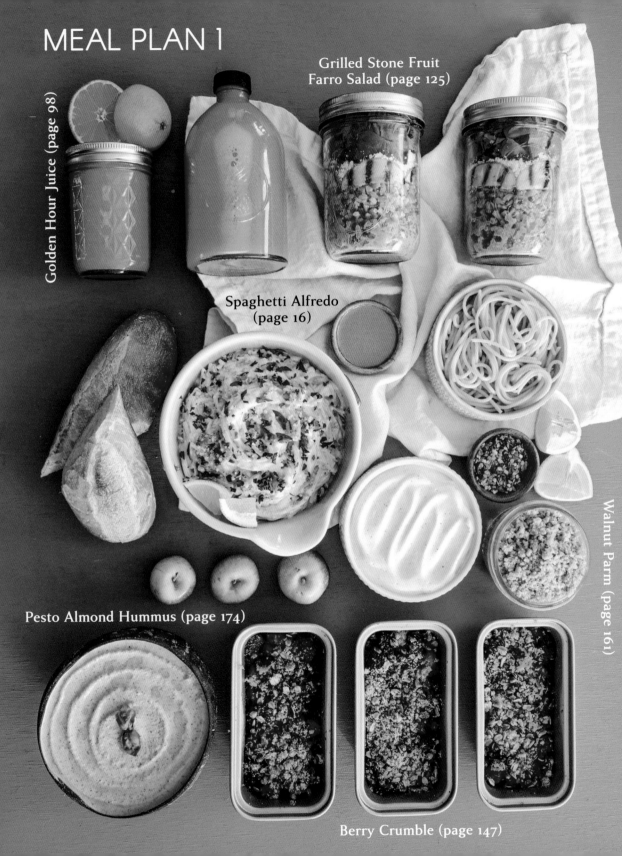

MEAL PLAN 1

Golden Hour Juice (page 98)

Grilled Stone Fruit
Farro Salad (page 125)

Spaghetti Alfredo
(page 16)

Walnut Parm (page 161)

Pesto Almond Hummus (page 174)

Berry Crumble (page 147)

BAI'S TIP: *Let the colors and produce of the seasons be your inspiration and guide through your meal prep and plant-based journey.*

MEAL PLAN 2

Go-To Green Juice (page 97)

Kale Caesar Salad (page 84)

Berrylicious Chia Jam (page 177)

Slightly Sweet Coconut Yogurt (page 169)

Chana Saag (page 41)

Pecan-Cacao Date Bars (page 144)

BAI'S TIP: Organize your meal prep around your work and exercise schedule. Plan your daily greens and plant-based protein just like you would a workout.

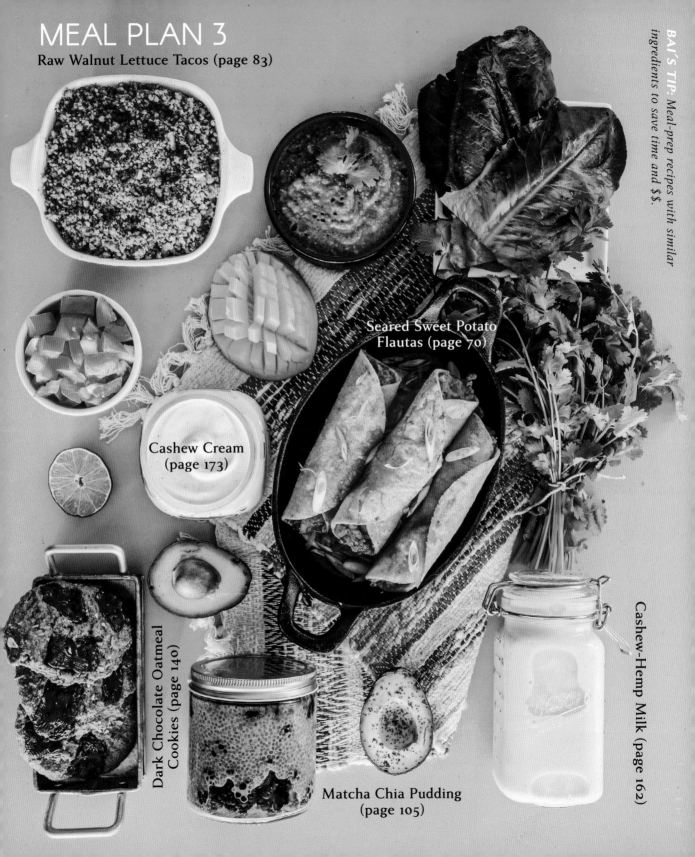

MEAL PLAN 3
Raw Walnut Lettuce Tacos (page 83)

BAI'S TIP: *Meal-prep recipes with similar ingredients to save time and $$.*

Seared Sweet Potato
Flautas (page 70)

Cashew Cream
(page 173)

Dark Chocolate Oatmeal
Cookies (page 140)

Matcha Chia Pudding
(page 105)

Cashew-Hemp Milk (page 162)

Acknowledgments

To my husband, Steve: You were there for me in my sickest hour. You took me to countless doctors, to surgery, and through it all, you never festered. You held me, helped me take my life back and dove into this mission right alongside me. Because of you, I had the courage to go vegan in all aspects of life and business. You have showed compassion, patience and love in a way I'd never experienced before. Thank you for being there and for believing in a better future for all of us. I am a better person because of you.

To my mom: You're the one who's been there through it all. You always taught me to never settle for anything less than what sets my soul on fire. Thank you for always answering the phone, talking me off the cliff and being the sounding board for my life. Your love for life and very convincing way to celebrate even the smallest wins has made this process unforgettable.

To my dad: My Yankee! You taught me to never accept anything less than what I deserve, and you taught me a work ethic that helped me get through the late nights of cooking, retesting recipes and writing. Your no-BS attitude on life has taught me to expect more from the world around us and to always strive to be better. Thanks for giving me thick skin and the sass to match.

Travis: You filmed my first cooking show when I was eight and have been my cheering squad ever since. It's no mistake we ended up in each other's lives again when I was writing this book. Your encouragement and daily banter made the process of writing this book a time I will never forget.

Paulina: My culinary soul sister and culinary school bestie. You gave me the courage to go vegan all those years ago when I thought you were totally crazy for doing it. Your dedication to yourself, your craft and your family has inspired me since the moment we met as a couple of kids in culinary school. Although our lives are far apart now, I felt you so much while writing this book.

The Chef Bai community: You all are amazing. Because of you, this work was possible. Your attendance to our classes, your re-creations of my recipes and your boundless support is something I could have only dreamed of. Thank you for showing up for us and for yourselves in the process. Love you so big!

The Page Street Publishing team and Sarah: Thank you for believing in my work. Thank you for taking a chance on a first-time author and for working so hard to get this book published. None of it would be possible without you, and I am so grateful!

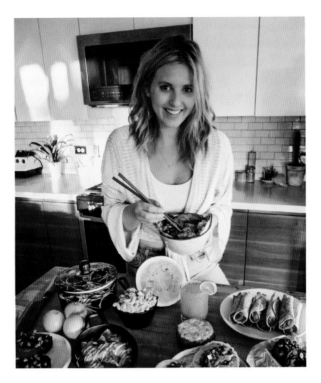

About the Author

BAILEY RUSKUS (A.K.A. CHEF BAI) is a plant-based professional chef and culinary instructor originally from Boulder, Colorado. She graduated from Le Cordon Bleu in San Francisco and pursued further education at the Institute for Integrative Nutrition and the T. Colin Campbell Center for Nutrition Studies. She has taught thousands of people around the world the power of healing through food. Chef Bai has also cooked for and worked with all different kinds of people, from bestselling authors and corporate companies to the everyday family, community initiatives and nonprofits. She has been cooking professionally and internationally since 2010. She is now the host of her own podcast (*The Plant Remedy*) while she runs her business, and is a voice for environmental and animal activism. Chef Bai's main focuses are corporate wellness initiatives, corporate brand recipe development, community cooking classes and online cooking and healing programs. If you would like to reach out to Chef Bai, head to www.chefbai.kitchen to join her online membership or get in contact.

Index

Avocado Curry Noodles, 45

Breakfast Tacos with Ranchero Sauce, 113

Cauliflower-Avocado Ceviche, 56

Chilaquiles, 77

Crispy Carnitas Mushroom Burritos, 66

Mediterranean Veggie Skewers with Chimichurri, 88

Seared Sweet Potato Flautas and Avocado Salsa Verde, 70

Tacos Al Pastor, 61-62

K

kale

Curried Coconut Lentil Salad, 122

Kale Caesar Salad, 84

Roasted Sweet Potatoes with Crispy Kale and Tahini Dressing, 90-91

Rustic Italian Chopped Salad, 130

Kale Caesar Salad, 84

kidney beans, in Hibiscus Taco Salad, 73

kimchi, in Crispy Tofu Rainbow Bali Bowl, 133

L

lasagna noodles, in Roasted Red Pepper Lasagna, 19

leeks

Flaky, Buttery Biscuits and Mushroom Gravy, 33-34

Immune-Boosting Veggie Broth, 170

Moroccan Lentil Soup, 137

lentils

Curried Coconut Lentil Salad, 122

Flaky, Buttery Biscuits and Mushroom Gravy, 33-34

Moroccan Lentil Soup, 137

Polenta with Spicy Tomato Chorizo, 69

lettuce

Go-To Green Juice, 97

Raw Walnut Lettuce Tacos, 83

lime juice

Breakfast Tacos with Ranchero Sauce, 113

Cauliflower-Avocado Ceviche, 56

Crispy Carnitas Mushroom Burritos, 66

Crispy Tofu Rainbow Bali Bowl, 133

Hibiscus Taco Salad, 73

Jackfruit Tortilla Soup, 65

Seared Sweet Potato Flautas and Avocado Salsa Verde, 70

Tacos Al Pastor, 61-62

limes

Mediterranean Veggie Skewers with Chimichurri, 88

Polenta with Spicy Tomato Chorizo, 69

Raw Walnut Lettuce Tacos, 83

Seared Sweet Potato Flautas and Avocado Salsa Verde, 70

Tacos Al Pastor, 61-62

Watermelon Poke Bowls, 42

M

Mac 'n' Cheesy Goodness, 23

mangos

Chia Pudding Three Ways, 105

Crispy Tofu Rainbow Bali Bowl, 133

Raw Walnut Lettuce Tacos, 83

Tacos Al Pastor, 61-62

The Vibrant Roll, 126

Tropical Green Smoothie, 102

Meal Plans, 181-183

Mediterranean Veggie Skewers with Chimichurri, 88

micro greens, in Chilaquiles, 77

Midnight Dream Smoothie, 101

Miso-Mushroom Ramen, 38

Mocha Chocolate Cake with Avocado Frosting, 154-155

Mole Family-Style Enchiladas, 59-60

Moroccan Lentil Soup, 137

mozzarella cheese, in Roasted Red Pepper Lasagna, 19

mung beans, in The Ultimate Breakfast Sando, 119

mushrooms

Breakfast Tacos with Ranchero Sauce, 113-115

Chicago-Style Classic Deep-Dish Pizza, 51-52

Chilaquiles, 77

Crispy Carnitas Mushroom Burritos, 66

Flaky, Buttery Biscuits and Mushroom Gravy, 33-34

Mediterranean Veggie Skewers with Chimichurri, 88

Miso-Mushroom Ramen, 38

Polenta with Spicy Tomato Chorizo, 69